Sweats, Frets but no Regrets

An insider's guide to the Menopause

Dr L. D. Taylor

Disclaimer

The information contained in this book is provided for general purposes only. It is not intended as and should not be relied upon as medical advice. The author is not responsible for any specific health needs that may require medical supervision. If you have underlying health problems or have any doubts about the advice contained in this book, you should contact a qualified medical or other appropriate professional.

This book details the author's personal experiences with and opinions about the menopause. The author is not your healthcare provider and this information is not designed to diagnose, treat, prevent or cure any condition and is for information purposes only.

The author is providing this book and its contents on an "as is" basis, all areas of medicine are subject to change and new research findings. The author does not represent or warrant that the information accessible via this book is accurate, complete or current. The author will not be liable for damages arising out of or in connection with the use of this book.

This book provides content related to physical and mental health issues. Use of this book implies your acceptance of this disclaimer.

References are provided for informational purposes only and do not constitute endorsement of any websites or other sources.

Introduction

It's a funny thing being a female doctor, you can map your own ageing to the increasing age of the women you see in your clinics. I went from being the 'little baby doctor' (so named by the elderly ladies in the local warden assisted housing) who was seeing young women seeking contraception and sexual health advice, to being the doctor sought out for the menopause.

Whilst I offered my best care by keeping up to date and ensuring I knew as much as I could about this subject, it wasn't until I travelled the flush-ridden, sleep-deprived journey myself that I was truly able to consult with empathy.

I went through my menopause at forty-four and it hurt. I was lucky not to have much change in my periods, they simply stopped; but I was suddenly hot (and not in the pin-up sort of way) and grumpy and tired and anxious...and believe you me, these were not usual states for me.

I was in the fortunate position of knowing what this was. I didn't have a bunch of horrible illnesses and I wasn't developing a psychiatric diagnosis. In short, having the knowledge that this is what the menopause could cause, put me, I believe, in a stronger position to ride it out and, where able, do something to lessen the effects.

For so long the menopause has been a little-discussed subject, the symptoms might be considered embarrassing or private and it's not been a natural water cooler topic; in fact, the menopausal women at the watercooler are the ones with their foreheads pressed against it, unable to talk at all.

Thankfully, in the past few years the menopause has started to make its way into popular culture, which in turn makes it easier to talk about and embrace.

Who wouldn't want to be Kristin Scott Thomas' effortlessly cool menopausal character in Fleabag? And whilst our cartoons stay stationary in time, can you imagine fast-forwarding Marge Simpson's heaven-scraping blue hair to a menopausal sweat fest?

7

I've been pretty talkative about my menopause from the start, mainly because I can't bear to suffer in silence and I need everyone to share my pain; but also because, as a doctor, I hadn't realised that there were rules. It wasn't until I was at an 80th birthday party, chatting to the somewhat older lady next to me and making a usual-for-me menopause jibe (menopause brain? Menopause belly? Menopause attempting to destroy my life?) and for her to look at me as if I was sharing my toileting habits, that I realised that's not generally how it's done.

I also realised that despite the increase in information available, you do have to know what you're looking for, and if you simply don't know that the symptom you're suffering from may be related to the menopause, then how do you know what to do next?

This really came home to me when I was chatting with girlfriends (with wine - beware, wine becomes the menopausal woman's poison) and I fleetingly complained (did I mention I was gabby on this subject?) that the worst thing I'd experienced with my menopause to date was the anxiety. Three of my non-medical friends

chimed in with '...What? Anxiety? Is that a menopause thing? Wow, I'm so relieved to hear that...' and out came all their stories.

I was surprised because:

> A. I surround myself with clever women (so some of their glory rubs off on me) and

> B. My only real experience of women going through the menopause to date, were those who'd sought me out in clinic, so were already part-way on the journey to understanding that something was changing and had already done a little research and information checking.

I thought I'd like to do something to share the knowledge and the love, maybe a quick-fire information book/audio/vlog about my journey; that was five years ago now (menopausal fatigue anyone?). The mind was willing but the body and brain were significantly less caught up with the plan.

Here we finally are though.

I realised a vlog was simply too millennial for me, I want you to know this stuff, but I'm not too worried about you knowing me; and more honestly, my marionette and empathy (!) brow lines do not stand up to close video inspection. (In fact, do all smartphone/tablet makers have shares in Botox? There seems to be nothing more ageing than being reflected back in one; it makes you want to scurry off to the nearest clinic to be jabbed. Thank goodness for reflective make up and for Zoom and all their crazy filters...although I've some way to go before I start appearing in meetings as a cat...)

So, I've gone with the book/audiobook option. I've split this book into bite sized chunks so you can fast track to the anxiety chapter or the weight one without having to look under the car bonnet at the facts and physiology if that's not your thing.

I'll repeat a few messages within each chapter (which will be a bit annoying if you're reading it from front to back – so apologies in advance for that). I loathe a self-help book that simply rehashes the same story in twenty different ways, so please feedback if there is too much repetition and I'll cut some out for version 2. (get me, getting ahead of myself!)

I've done a lot of reading for this book. Actually that's not true, I've done a lot of reading for myself which has made it into this book. I will list some of the authors and papers that you may wish to seek out yourself. I've created a set of resources which you can use to take you to the next level of understanding.

I'm not going to attempt to find all the answers for you. To be honest, within this foray, I'd really just like you to know what's happening; because I think knowing what's happening is the real starting point for being able to take charge and feel in control. I'll give you a few tips, arm you with the facts and give you a stronger base to decide what to do next.

Right, let's get to it. The Menopause 101. Let's make it yours - understand it, own it.

And then, if you're currently in a relationship, hand it over to your partner to read; believe me, you're going to need them on board and this is probably the quickest way to achieve that.

What is the menopause?

OK - dry chapter warning!

So, what is the menopause? It is simply a date in the diary, it is the point where you have not had a period for 12 months. The median age for the menopause in the UK and US for instance is 51 yrs old.

Perimenopause is the time during which you have symptoms but haven't yet gone a full year without a period (you may hear it referred to as the climacteric too). Many women will get symptoms up to four or five years before their last period and they can continue for many years after.

So we have the perimenopause (the symptomatic phase up to the last period + twelve months), the menopause and thereafter you're postmenopausal; which makes it sound as though it's all over but believe me, it's not!

You're probably thinking 'who cares', but in fact, these dates are important e.g. if you started bleeding post-menopausally, we would investigate this, but bleeding before this is to be expected. In fact, many women can go months without a bleed and then have two or three months of regular bleeding before they stop again; that full year without a bleed is crucial for diagnosis. (Abnormal bleeding patterns are something different and we'll come to those later.)

In addition to that, another way we categorize the menopause is in relation to what age you are when you go through it. This is important because it affects contraception advice and also what extra risks you may be exposed to if you go through an early menopause.

If you're under the age of 40 and have had twelve months without a period, this isn't called the menopause, but Premature Ovarian Insufficiency and that's a whole different ball game. It's something that doctors would want to know about sooner than a year - about four to six months in fact, depending on which health care system you live within - as we would investigate this further and maybe refer you onwards for advice; so that's something that you don't simply go through at home.

Age 40 to 45yrs is called *early* menopause.

45yrs and above - all good, you're just straightforward menopausal, no special qualifiers.

The final way to qualify the menopause is natural vs not. How can a menopause not be natural you're wondering; well, if you have your ovaries removed then this is a surgical menopause and rather than waiting the full twelve months to qualify for your badge, you are handed it immediately.

There are also drugs e.g. chemotherapy, and illnesses that can lead to a stoppage of periods but this can tend to be a bit erratic so in some cases you may need to wait the full twelve months again before being sure. (This is one of those 'check in with your oncologist/doctor' moments.)

So what's happening and why is it happening?

I was really pleased, when I was doing my reading, to discover that whilst other animals do go through a menopause, only a few share women's ability to remain alive many years post-menopause.

Most women will survive three decades after their menopause and so do orca, beluga and short-finned pilot whales plus a few insects (but let's gloss over those.)

There were times when I hit peak weight gain that I shared plenty more characteristics with whales than my ability to live beyond my reproductive years. Greenpeace sightings of pilot whales off the south coast of England stood down on realising that it was just me, post-menopausal kitesurfer, hitting the shorebreak.

The simplest version of what's happening is that your ovaries are ageing and the amount of hormones that they produce are reducing until they stop producing them altogether.

The usual menstrual cycle is a beautiful dance of hormone increases and decreases, each interacting with the other; this now becomes a bit of a free for all and the levels are fluctuating without following the old rules - think of it as a transition from waltzing to pogo-ing.

Over a period of time you go from 100% oestrogen to < 1% because apart from a small amount produced by the adrenal gland and some produced in our adipose (fat) cells, the ovary is the main power house. The ovary also produces a hormone called progesterone, and to a lesser extent testosterone and these are reducing too.

Interestingly, oestrogen can remain within normal range for much of the perimenopause but it's the fluctuation of these hormone levels that causes so many of the symptoms.

Generally, as doctors, we don't do much in terms of blood testing for investigating the perimenopause unless you have other symptoms that don't fit or seem excessive e.g. joint swelling in addition to joint pain. Not all symptoms at this age are menopause, although it can often feel like that.

Essentially if you're over 45 and you're getting a number of symptoms that are strongly perimenopausal, then it's a clinical diagnosis. There are symptom trackers and also a Climacteric Symptom scale which can be helpful for supporting this clinical diagnosis. I really recommend using a symptom tracker as you can also start learning about triggers (which we'll also come to later) and I'll pop a recommendation or two on the resource sheet.

If you're 40 to 45, then your doctor may run a few blood tests: the marker FSH (follicle stimulating hormone) can be helpful for supporting a diagnosis, although less so if you're still having periods; however FSH is no help at all if you're on some types of hormonal medication e.g. the combined oral contraceptive pill.

Women who've had a hysterectomy but still have their ovaries may go through the menopause earlier than average (this is thought to be to do with the changes to the blood flow post-op) and again, doctors tend to simply accept the symptoms as confirmation but may offer a blood test for surety.

For those who are interested I have put a link to learn more about the normal physiology of the cycle; given that it is such a precision cycle, you can see how if one thing goes out of kilter that can have an impact on something else e.g. the bleeding pattern.

Right let's move on to the symptoms...

Symptoms - the good, the bad and the unexpected

How many of us will experience symptoms, what are they and how do you recognise them for what they are?

Well, be reassured you're not alone. Up to 80% of women will be affected by the symptoms of the menopause. You will undoubtedly have a pal who will race through it without even breaking a sweat, but you can see from the number above that they're in the minority. You do get close to wanting to put their friendship on hold until you've emerged out the other side but pretend I didn't say that out loud.

Let's look at them.

Whilst the idea of a long list doesn't really lend itself to the audiobook format, there is something quite nice about glancing down and seeing your symptom. It's OK! You're in the club, you're on the list, there may be a reason for you feeling so wretched.

And do you know what? This is a good club to be in. Both ayurvedic medicine and yoga recognise the postmenopausal time as a period of wisdom and grace. Sometimes it can just feel really difficult to get your hands on that grace when you're sweating buckets and angry at everyone...at least angry at those whose names you can remember.

Doctors love to categorise symptoms according to body areas and I think that works here. For the visual of you, I've done a nice stick lady with a massive belly and lots of arrows pointing in an alarming way at various areas of her body to truly terrify.

So brace yourself, here's the main hitters, undoubtedly there will be more that I've forgotten but this is a starter for ten.

Nervous system (brain, spinal cord)

Hot flushes, flashes, power surges – call them what you will.

Night sweats

Difficulty sleeping

20

Racing heart (palpitations)

Memory loss

Brain fog

Reduced concentration

Headaches

Irritability

Anxiousness

Low mood

Emotional triggering

Mood swings

Muscles, bones and cartilage

Joint pains

Loss of muscle mass leading to weakness and tiring more easily

Changes in metabolism

Increased central weight gain (leading to insulin resistance)

Skin etc.

Dry skin (leading to itchiness)

Thinner, less elastic skin (wrinkles...let's call a spade a spade)

Dry eyes (leading to discomfort)

Dry mouth (leading to burning symptoms, and sometimes bleeding gums)

Hair loss (just when you're starting to get new hair on your chin...the menopause is very unkind!)

Gynae and waterworks (Genito-urinary system)

Change in bleeding pattern

Reduced sex drive

Pain with sex

Vaginal dryness, soreness, itching

Recurrent urine infections

Urinary frequency

Vaginal discharge

Urinary incontinence (losing urine involuntarily)

Gut

Constipation

Bloating (however not bloating that's present on waking)

Indigestion

Fatigue, absolute complete draining tiredness - 'lie on the bed and fall asleep even though you were meant to be just making it' fatigue

And the ones that you can't feel but are happening whether you like it or not

Bone thinning

Increased risk of heart disease

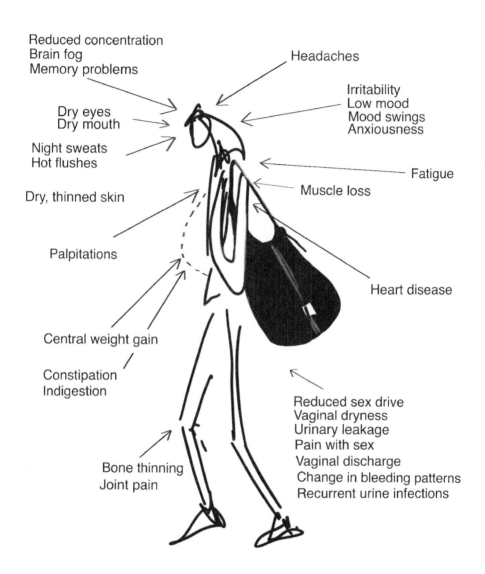

Reduced concentration
Brain fog
Memory problems

Headaches

Dry eyes
Dry mouth

Irritability
Low mood
Mood swings
Anxiousness

Night sweats
Hot flushes

Fatigue

Dry, thinned skin

Muscle loss

Palpitations

Heart disease

Central weight gain

Constipation
Indigestion

Reduced sex drive
Vaginal dryness
Urinary leakage
Pain with sex
Vaginal discharge
Change in bleeding patterns
Recurrent urine infections

Bone thinning
Joint pain

25

To be honest, when I was at the zenith of my perimenopause, it got to the point where it felt that the only thing I couldn't really blame on my menopause was my onychomycosis (which is a really fancy name for fungal toenail but I thought I'd try and spare you the horror of that vision...I do spend a lot of time in the water.)

It is a lot of symptoms and they're really diverse...oestrogen, the main player, is a hormone that you really only associate with your periods, so why on earth are you getting flushes and brain fog and crying all the time?

Oestrogen, progesterone and testosterone are essentially chemical messaging systems, and they can exert their action by being invited into an area via a doorway called a receptor. Anywhere that has an oestrogen receptor will be impacted by loss or changes in oestrogen. There are oestrogen receptors in places that you simply wouldn't think there would be e.g. the memory centre of the brain, so you can see why the above list is so lengthy.

In addition to this way of working, researchers are now finding that oestrogen can work by supporting other chemical messengers to create a change so this extends its impact and thus the symptoms you might see when it's not present.

There are also what I call the 'vicious circle symptoms'; you sweat which makes you sleep badly which in turn causes you to gain more central abdominal fat which might cause you to start snoring, this will affect your sleep quality and lead to poor sleep which in turn makes you want to eat more sugar...see where I'm going here?

Or, you find sex painful once, which makes you anxious that the next time you have sex it will also be painful, and so you keep putting it off, which makes your partner worried and then you feel anxious as they seem more distant and you sleep less well as you're worrying about your relationship, so you gain more weight and you sweat more and you think why would anyone want to have sex with you when you're overweight and sweaty to boot...Dramatic? Me?

Do you see what I mean? Because each of these symptoms touches on all parts of our living, it is easy to get caught in a downward spiral.

In addition to the above you are dealing with :

A loss – the menopause marks the end of our ability to reproduce, and this can have a huge emotional impact. It is a milestone of ageing, we've got our big birthdays but there is no denying this crossing from one side to another is significant and not shared by men. It can feel like a very lonely place to stand.

It's also happening at a time that is often jam packed with life changes, if you have children they may be leaving home, your parents may have hit an age when they require a lot of support, you may have just missed a promotion at work, you may be questioning your role in the world...

There have been a couple of surveys in recent years run by the British Menopause society which have looked at symptoms and women's experience of them.

Some low moments for me were knowing that so many women were simply suffering in silence.

BMS survey 2016

- *'...50% of women aged 45-65 who have experienced the menopause in the last ten years hadn't consulted a healthcare professional about their symptoms*

- *This despite the fact that women report an average of seven symptoms and 42% feel their menopause symptoms were worse/much worse than expected...'*

Also, (and this goes back to my original reason for trying for another way to get the information out there), many women reported experiencing symptoms that they hadn't expected e.g. disturbed sleep, memory and concentration problems.

Here's a few more choice findings:

- 79% had hot flushes

- 70% had night sweats

- 50% said it impacted on their home life

- 36% said it impacted on their social life

- 50% said it impacted on their sex life

Ok, I'm making myself feel sad now so let's crack on and start talking about some of these symptoms in more detail and where able, offer a few tips for how to keep them at bay; if you like wine, you're not going to like one of those tips.

The so-called Vasomotor symptoms

Ok, flushes, sweats and palpitations...in a word - grim.

Flushes and sweats - 70% to 80% of women suffer from them and they're probably the symptoms we most associate with the menopause. So, what are they?

Well, first let me tell you what they feel like; they feel like a horrible little gremlin is firing up a camping stove inside you. You get very hot, usually over the face, chest and head, often your skin flushes red, and you may or may not sweat profusely, and then when it's over, you go all cold and clammy. Glorious.

The thing about this gremlin is that they don't light this stove at a time when you might need it, for example when you're walking out in a snow storm. No, that would be way too useful, instead they light it at the most inappropriate moments...

Let's imagine your pal who's recently divorced, she's got all her brave tokens together and has decided to try dating again, she's off to meet someone for a nice cup of coffee, and she's feeling a little bit stressed. So while she's sitting waiting for her date to arrive, BANG, the flush hits.

Her beautifully crafted make up is now sliding down her face, her hair is plastered to her cheeks and she's gone a bright puce...way to bring that carefully built up confidence crashing back down to the ground.

Ooh and did I mention that her heart might start racing and she's probably feeling a bit nauseated and light headed? These are the other vasomotor symptoms associated with the menopause.

Other good times for the sweats to turn up - you're just about to present at a meeting, or at a 'I so want this job' interview, or when you're applying for grant funding from the Dean at the university (fortunately she's female, so gets it). Yup, not when needed to reduce the heating bills but most often at really, really inconvenient times.

Some women will get a few a week, others will be swamped by them. They tend to turn up more at night so in turn lead to disrupted sleep. Supposedly they last, on average, four minutes (I did not know this until I found it written in a zillion places), it feels like much longer and for some women it is. They can continue for anything up to fifteen years after the menopause although this is unusual. The average time with flushes is about two years.

You'll notice a lot of the situations I've mentioned above are times that we might be nervous, and this is important. Flushes can often be triggered by certain things including feeling anxious or stressed. Learning your triggers can be helpful for at least reducing flushes, although it's unlikely to stop them completely.

So let's quickly check in on what's happening (or skip right on past) and then we'll head to the triggers.

The area in the brain called the hypothalamus regulates temperature; oestrogen has a direct effect on this part of the brain and also on a set of chemicals called neurotransmitters.

Whilst it's not been established exactly what causes menopausal flushes, it's thought that with the changing levels of oestrogen, the temperature regulation becomes faulty and the hypothalamus acts as if the body is too hot and tries to reduce the core temperature by sending more blood to the outskirts to cool down. This is achieved by widening our veins...which you can see as flushing of the skin and feel as heat.

The other way the body naturally cools down (think of what happens on a hot day) is to sweat; as the sweat evaporates from the body, it takes heat with it. These are normal physiological responses to being too hot, but they're now happening at random.

Flushes and sweats are not just the province of the menopausal woman. They can be associated with some drugs and also some illnesses e.g. an overactive thyroid and some infections like TB can also present with sweats.

Also lots of people, not just menopausal ones, can sweat and flush when they eat spicy food or drink alcohol. There is much to be said for checking in at least once with your doctor to ensure that we're all talking about the same thing.

Smokers get more flushes than non smokers, and there is an association between a higher blood sugar and more flushes too. This is an area that's attracting a lot of attention at the moment, as researchers try to unpick which symptoms and chemical changes may be associated with the increased incidence of heart disease in post-menopausal women. Something we'll come to later.

In terms of triggers, this is where a symptom tracker really comes into its own as whilst there's a list of things that are generally thought to worsen flushes, there are going to be some of those that may not be a problem for you and there may be triggers that you find that no one else gets.

Here's a few:

- Alcohol (aaaarrrrgggghhhh hhhhh!)

- Caffeine (crying inside...)

- Moving from one temperature environment to another

- Spicy foods

- Eating or drinking piping hot food

- Feeling anxious/stressed (lots of chemicals rushing around playing havoc with your systems)

<u>What can you do to try and reduce their frequency?</u>

I'm going to talk about lifestyle stuff here but at the end of the book, I'll pop links to sites with information about medications or supplements that can be taken.

Some of this will seem barn door obvious but sometimes you have to see it written down to realise. Lots of this isn't 'science' based but things that women have told me over the years that have worked for them, things I had to do myself and then of course the scientists' excellent offerings.

- Avoid the above list (;-))...OK, I appreciate that's a really annoying bullet point

- Wear layers - I am the queen of the layer, I will start with a light no-sleeve top and then it's easy to add and remove layers. I also find that natural fibres work best: viscose, merino, bamboo for example.

- Consider two single duvets if you share the bed (a friend of mine has a silk duvet...how luxurious does that sound?)

- Keep your bedroom cool (this is good for sleep even if you're not menopausal)

- Sip cool drinks through the day

- Use a handheld fan (I have to say, I've never managed this...I can't help but strike an overly dramatic pose)

- Have lukewarm showers or baths rather than hot ones

- Cool spritz for the face or cool gel pack (you might be able to offset a flush by a quick spray and an iced drink...everything's worth a try)

- Meditation

More science-based long-term investment to reduce frequency:

- Exercise regularly

- Give up smoking

- Cognitive behaviour therapy

- Reduce central weight gain

- Keep blood sugar regulated

More on these in later chapters.

So even I'm a bit annoyed by this listing of things, let's go back to that first example...what could our imaginary dating friend do to try and reduce the chance of that debilitating flush?

Arrive early. The change in temperature from outside to in may trigger a hot flush so she's got time to get half undressed when she arrives and redressed (if she fancies) before they turn up.

She could do a breathing practice before leaving the house or whilst waiting for her date to arrive (BTW if they're more than ten minutes late with no communication to say why, then let's tell our imaginary friend to leave. That's not menopause advice but just ensuring our pal doesn't end up dating a waste of space; life's too short to spend on people who don't value you right from the outset.)

She could avoid SPF make up (generally wear it, but not in the evenings or for one off dates inside. Go mineral instead).

She should layer her clothing so she can divest and add according to where she's at on the flushometer. (I'd always wondered why so many middle aged women wear those throw pashmina-y things, and now I know.)

Choose an airy cafe and sit near an open window or outside (under an umbrella).

Order a cool iced drink...not alcohol or coffee or iced tea.

If she eats - then she should let the food sit and cool some, and avoid ordering anything with chilli or paprika.

Bonne chance, good luck, etc. tell me where you're going and text when you're home - I won't judge.

I can't think therefore I no longer am

You'd think as a doctor that I'd know all the places that you can find an oestrogen or progesterone receptor (the doorway to let a hormone into a part of a cell to do its work) but I have to admit when I was reading the nattily named 'Cognition, Mood and Sleep in Menopausal transition' review paper, I got a few surprises...they seem to be sprinkled around the brain like fairy dust.

They're found in the parts of the brain that control memory and also the areas in charge of 'executive function' - this is the air traffic controller bit of the brain that allows us to overlook a thousand distracting messages whilst making decisions, to plan, prioritise and also to exercise a bit of self control (second piece of chocolate cake anyone?).

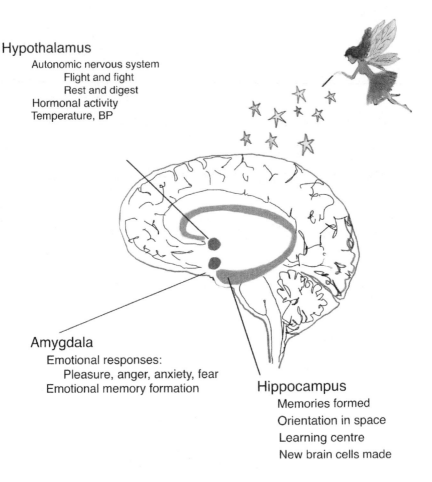

Hypothalamus
Autonomic nervous system
Flight and fight
Rest and digest
Hormonal activity
Temperature, BP

Amygdala
Emotional responses:
Pleasure, anger, anxiety, fear
Emotional memory formation

Hippocampus
Memories formed
Orientation in space
Learning centre
New brain cells made

Oestrogen additionally is thought to help the powerhouses of the brain cells, mitochondria, use energy more efficiently (and the brain uses a lot of energy). It improves the health of the cells making them more robust and less likely to be damaged, which is an effect shared by progesterone too.

As mentioned later in the sleep chapter, progesterone also works within one of the pathways in the brain (the GABA pathway) and can produce an anti-anxiety effect. More work is coming through to show that the reduction in testosterone does have an impact on brain function too.

Given all those receptors and the fact that those three hormones all have an effect on the brain, it will come as no surprise that when you go through the menopause and these hormones are all over the shop, that that is going to have an impact on how you feel and how you think. Hence the brain fog (that feeling that your brain has turned into candy floss and you simply can't make a decision), the difficulty with word finding, the reduced memory and also the anxiousness, low mood and emotional ups and downs.

In addition to this direct impact of oestrogen and progesterone, we might not be sleeping well and that also has an effect on memory, problem solving and mood.

This is so much worse for those who've had a surgical menopause. The going from truly 100% oestrogen to nearly zero overnight is the menopause X 100. Research shows significant obvious changes to memory reduction and verbal fluency whereas that's not quite so convincing in the research for the rest of us perimenopause types. We're lucky (really!) as our levels fluctuate over a period of time and some parts of the brain start taking up the slack and setting up their own systems to make up for this loss.

I used to be someone who could remember a name after one telling, I could carry my diary around in my head, I'd read something once and it would be mine. During this time I found myself in a position where I felt unable to trust my memory and this flowed over into work and play. I was constantly rechecking my decisions - throw a little snifter of anxiety into the mix and before you know it, your job is taking double or triple the time.

Patients and friends were telling me about situations where they'd been giving a presentation and come to a standstill, or couldn't remember their boss's name; or where previously they'd been really engaged at meetings, they were now too worried to give an opinion as they might forget what they wanted to say halfway through.

Here's some findings from another British Menopause Society survey, this time run in 2017:

- 45% of women felt that the menopause had had a negative impact on their work

- 47% who had needed to take a day off because of menopause symptoms said that they wouldn't tell employers the reason

This can be crippling in the workplace and at home. We define ourselves by so many things and for lots of us being good at our job is pretty high on that list.

Reassuringly it is thought that this time will settle, even for our surgical menopause pals; the SWAN study reported a reduction in learning abilities during the menopause but these did seem to return to usual ageing after time.

Quite wonderfully, and entirely news to me, certain areas in the brain can make oestrogen when the ovaries' supply has come to a standstill; this is used directly in the brain cell itself or locally in nearby cells, so wouldn't, for example, show up on a blood test. Undoubtedly an area for longer term study.

There does seem to be a movement to ensure that employers understand this time better (the British Medical Association did a survey on female doctors and their experience of the menopause last year). Women in turn should feel able to speak to a line manager about their experiences, or if you're the CEO then look at the business and work out how you might support women within it whilst cutting yourself a bit of slack.

It may be that working more flexibly will help. Working from home is now part of our daily routine with Covid and so there is an opportunity to control your work environment. Now, for example, you don't need to fall out with the rest of the office when you want the air conditioner on 5 degrees in the middle of winter.

It may be that we have to accept that we can't do it all, all of the time. Ask for longer to do tasks, (we'll still do them brilliantly, we are women after all) or find an opportunity to come back after meetings with ideas.

If you're at home with the children juggling family life, you may need to consider putting that SuperMum epithet to the side for a while and offer up the occasional shop-bought meal and cut out the third after-school club taxi ride. You'll still be SuperMum to us.

Let's not allow this to be another area to beat ourselves up and let's talk about it a bit more and be kind to our temporarily stalled brain.

Try to get your sleep sorted (coming to this soon), reduce those triggers for flushes (it's impossible to concentrate on anything whilst your pulse is racing and your hair is wet) and be gentle with yourself.

Recognise your internal voice when it starts taking you down a path of anxiety and self blame and bring it to a halt. This is happening to pretty much every woman of your age, and guess what? If the testosterone reduction is affecting our brain, then it will be affecting our male colleagues' brains too (their testosterone levels drop as they age) and I bet they're not holding themselves to task on it!

Good things happen post menopause - Ruth Bader Ginsburg was 60 yrs old when she was elected to the Supreme Court and she stayed there working until her death at age 87 yrs. Makes me feel knackered thinking about it, but what a woman!

Collagen - chicken neck anyone?

Before we go on to the changes to the skin, eyes, joints and bones, it's probably worth taking a moment to talk about collagen...which I do admit, does sound like something of a dull diversion.

This is a protein and has a bunch of different subtypes but the 1-3 are probably the most represented with 4 and 5 popping along behind and a whole bunch of others making small appearances.

Here's some of the places you'll find it:

Skin

Bone

Cartilage

Ligaments, Tendons

Cornea of the eye

Blood vessels

Teeth

Muscles

And more...

What does collagen do? It's an architectural building block, a long fibre that acts as support to hold things together, as a skeleton to add other proteins/minerals to e.g. bone is collagen with minerals added, and as a cover to provide protection.

Your body is in charge of making its own collagen - the building blocks are glycine and proline which are found in meat, fish, eggs, dairy, some legumes and tofu. Vitamin C and copper are involved in the pathway too and are found in your citrus, leafy veg, whole grains and nuts. I found this nutrition bit out by typing 'how do we get collagen into our lives' into Ecosia...*other search engines do exist, etc.* This is not the sort of stuff you learn in med school.

Collagen reduces as we get older and not only does it reduce more in women than men, we also had less to start off with.

Oestrogen receptors have been found on fibroblasts which are the cells that make collagen and whilst it's not fully understood the role that oestrogen plays in the making collagen pathway, it is involved. Collagen in skin, for example, reduces by about 30% in the first few years after the menopause alongside that plummeting level of oestrogen.

You can see why I wanted to get that list out there. Lots of the symptoms of the menopause can be traced back to collagen e.g. joint pain and dry skin and I'm going on to talk about those now.

Bones, Muscles and Joints

OK, muscle, cartilage and bones in this chapter - not the most rockstar of the body systems but much more important than you might expect.

All of these areas are affected by normal ageing which is why we find the following problems in men as well as women. However, at the time of the menopause, there is an accelerated rate of both bone loss and muscle strength, which leaves women with a greater deficit and therefore at greater risk.

Bone

Bones are constantly on the move, not just as we waggle them around but also they are in a perpetual cycle of bone building and breaking down.

The building part of the process - osteoblastic bone formation if you'd like to get right into the nub of it - is more dominant until we hit about 30 yrs of age. Then the formation equals the breaking down (osteoclastic bone resorption) for a decade or so; then the process of loss starts to outrun the process of creation and our bones become thinner and less good quality.

Now this happens to everyone as part of ageing but in women there is a significantly increased loss during the first five years peri to post menopause. This then slows back to that of usual ageing, i.e. still losing but not so rapidly now. Osteoporosis (the bone thinning disease) is found in about 2% of 50 year old women and in about 50% of them by the time they reach 80.

Why does this matter? Thinner bones surely means lighter on the scales? Sadly, thinner bones mean weaker bones which means increased chance of fractures. Whilst the reduction in bone density and structural changes are occurring around the time of the menopause, we don't tend to see the fractures associated with this loss until mid 60's and onwards - the hip and wrist fractures and the reducing height seen with fractures in the spine.

Osteoporosis is the name of the disease associated with thinner, weaker bones and according to the WHO is diagnosed when the bone mineral density is significantly different (2 Standard deviations) from the norm.

However the problem is that the bone mineral density is only part of the change in osteoporosis, there is also a structural change that weakens the bones and makes them more likely to fracture. So the other part of the diagnosis is a retrospective one - i.e. you have a fragility fracture and then you get given the diagnosis.

What's a fragility fracture? One that happens '...following a fall from standing height or less...' although fractures in the spine '...may occur spontaneously, or as a result of routine activities such as bending or lifting....' (NICE guidelines). I've had a patient who was simply making her bed when she developed a fracture of the spine.

The numbers are phenomenal - in the UK there are 180,000 osteoporosis related fractures per year and 1 in 3 women will suffer from one or more in their lifetime.

You might be thinking 'well, they'll mend my hip fracture and I'll be back on my feet in no time' but sadly the consequences of hip fracture, for example, are far reaching.

NICE guidelines again '...About 50% of people with an osteoporotic fragility fracture of the hip can no longer live independently...Vertebral fractures can cause back pain, loss of height, and kyphosis. Severe kyphosis can lead to breathing difficulties; gastrointestinal problems (such as indigestion)...' (Kyphosis refers to the bending forward of the spine that you see in elderly people.)

Some women are even more at risk of osteoporosis:

- Low BMI (< 18.5) i.e. underweight - bone mineral density is one of the few places where having a high BMI partially protects against bone loss

- Excess alcohol drinkers

- Early menopause i.e. less than 45 yrs

- History of osteoporosis in an immediate relative, generally your Mum.

- Certain diseases e.g. Rheumatoid arthritis, coeliac disease

- Certain medications e.g. steroids

<u>What can you do?</u>

You can check to see what your risk is by doing your FRAX score. I've put a link to this in the resource sheet. It's something that's often offered within a well woman check but there's no reason at all why you can't do your own.

Ensure you enter the menopause with your best bone health - start that exercise now and if you have daughters, try to instill in them the idea that Amazonian beats waif hands down when it comes to body image.

Exercise

Some types of exercise can promote bone strength or at least prevent loss.

- Weight bearing exercise (walking, running, jumping, etc.) describes when your feet or arms are taking the entire weight of your body through them. When you exercise weight bearing, you are applying an impact or jolt to the skeleton which serves as a mechanical stimulus to the bone to promote bone making. Low impact force/stimulus= walking, high impact = star jumps. (Astronauts who float around in microgravity and therefore don't get weight bearing exercise can lose 1-2 % of their bone mass per month.)

- Weight or resistance training exercise - it's thought that when a muscle pulls on a bone during this type of exercise, it can stimulate bone growth but only in the muscle areas exercised.

- Balance exercises - these aren't going to have a direct effect on your bones but they will make it less likely that you'll fall over in the first place.

Give up smoking

Keep your alcohol intake within current guidelines.

Check your calcium intake - there are loads of calcium calculators online so you can check that your diet is providing enough. Check your local osteoporosis society guidelines for the amount recommended for post menopause, and for those with established osteoporosis. These numbers seem to differ across countries. A Cochrane study showed a very small increase in bone mineral density with 1000mg daily as an average dose.

Consider taking Vit D. In the UK the recommendation is to take Vit D from October through to April. This is because the majority of our Vit D comes from sun exposure and despite my self professed prune skin, we don't have enough of the good stuff over the winter in this country. (If you're reading this in California then I expect that's less of an issue). A small amount of Vit D comes from nutrition, it can be found in egg yolks, milk, meat and mushrooms to name a few.

Support your microbiome - this is all a bit brand new but there does seem to be work coming through linking a healthy microbiome to better bone health. I cover the microbiome in the gut chapter but I'm going to be keeping a close eye on this so will update via blog or Instagram as able.

Muscle

As mentioned men and women both lose muscle mass and strength as they age. This is impactful beyond simply not being able to open the coffee jar anymore; reduced muscle means that usual tasks are harder to do, and as a result we tire more quickly.

It's not entirely clear what role oestrogen plays in this but there is evidence of oestrogen receptors in muscle fibres and we know that it has an effect on the collagen which holds muscles together. Oestrogen also works with other chemicals like growth hormone and insulin growth factor at muscle level, and its loss means that those pathways become less effective.

A 65 - 80 year old woman can have double the amount of non - contractile muscle tissue compared with that of a 23 - 57 yr old (I love these random ages in Team 2). This sounds like we have bigger, better muscles; unfortunately it's the contractile muscle tissue that we want more of and now proportionally we have significantly less of that.

We've always stored fat in our muscles but now we're not so good at converting it into energy so it's just sitting there taking up valuable space. Muscle weighs more than fat so we may be the same weight when we jump on the scales and think that everything's fine in the world...but it's not, that's essentially a 'fat gain' not being recorded as a weight increase.

So why do we want more contractile or lean muscle mass?

- It burns fat cells - totally in love with this concept.

60

- It shares the work of the skeleton meaning we put less stress through our joints.

- It makes it easier to do tasks and therefore be less tired on completing them. If you walk up three flights of stairs every day for three weeks, at some point you don't even notice you're doing it and think quite happily about taking on the fourth. This is not simply cardiac conditioning, it is also because you're building more muscle in your legs to do this.

What can we do to prevent or at least reduce this reduction in contractile muscle tissue?

Exercise (eye rolling allowed!)

Exercise comes to the rescue once again. You may have noticed that magazines and blogs are talking more and more about resistance/weight training in women, and this is because it makes a difference over and above your usual cardio or endurance regime in this instance.

Weight training helps maintain muscle mass (everything is easier to maintain than it is to get back) and it reduces that intramuscular fat by using it directly as energy.

People doing resistance training have a greater muscle mass than endurance athletes e.g. marathon runners; human growth factor is released with exercise and it's thought more so with resistance training and this promotes muscle growth; so if you're a runner, it's worth adding some weight training (using weights, resistance bands, or lifting your own body weight e.g. push up, all count).

Nutrition

Nutrition comes down to making sure you're getting your protein on board. These are numbers that I'm sure gym bunnies know but they were news to me...0.8g per kilo of body weight is the amount of protein per day that is required to keep the balance between making muscle and breaking it down.

I'm not sure there are enough hours in the day for me to start working out how much protein I'm getting per meal but I guess if I started finding walking up stairs a chore, I might consider it.

Vit D

There are Vit D receptors on muscle and people who have a Vit D level in the higher part of the normal range have been found to have better physical performance scores. Vit D deficiency can show up as muscle and bone pain, muscle weakness and fatigue.

Joints

And now on to those aching joints.

The joints have cartilage lining them and as we know cartilage is made of collagen and we also know that oestrogen has a direct effect on the production of collagen.

Losing our muscle mass means that our joints are under more stress as muscles share the load of weight bearing with the joints.

We're gaining weight so this also is putting more pressure on the joints.

There's a term called 'climacteric arthralgia' which is a fancy name for the joint pain we see at the menopause. Mine particularly affected the small joints of my hands and feet, and my lower back started playing up. It was worse in the morning and it took me about ten minutes to unwind my spine and get upright when it was at its worst.

It is uncomfortable and sort of surprising. This was definitely one of those symptoms that had me querying menopause vs other? One of my friends also developed painful joints around this time however hers were secondary to an inflammatory arthritis, so it's worth a check in to be sure that you don't have any signs/symptoms that fit with this.

What lifestyle treatments do we have for this?

- Lose weight if you're overweight

- Build more muscle to share the load

- Diet and microbiome may have an impact here too; there's information linking diet to inflammatory arthritis but I've not found anything directly about the microbiome and menopause joint pain but I'll share when/if I do!

Skin, Hair, Eyes and Mouth

Skin

Ooh, just as I finish writing this a friend of a friend has published a book about the skin changes involved with the different ages of life, so for specific information about what to do best at the perimenopause, I shall direct you there in the resource sheet.

After offering a little glowing light of support, let me lower your mood by describing the skin changes that occur at the time of the menopause and then try to find ways to brighten you back up again by sharing a few dietary offerings.

Age causes skin changes regardless of whether you're passing through the menopause or not, so therefore in order to work out what's oestrogen related and what's not, the research mostly looks at women taking hormone replacement therapy, compared with age/lifestyle matched women who aren't.

Oestrogen affects the skin in a number of ways - it has a direct effect on elastin, collagen, the blood supply to the skin and promotes good wound healing.

Without oestrogen, elastin is reduced; as its name suggests this plays a part in the skin's elasticity; this loss leads to wrinkling and dryness.

The levels of collagen in the skin reduce significantly, and given that collagen forms the major component of skin, not unsurprisingly loss causes skin to become and look thinner.

The amount of blood that gets to the skin is also reduced and healing from wounds is less good.

According to one review paper I read, collagen types 1 and 3 decrease by as much as 30% in the first five years post-menopause. This is up there with the amount of bone loss that can occur in the immediate years post menopause; which makes sense given that collagen is the base structural protein for bone too.

When you look at skin depth in elderly women, thinner skin appears to be related more to the years they spent without oestrogen than chronological age and interestingly women with osteoporotic fractures have thinner skin.

You've probably noticed that there is a golden age when you can't really tell the difference between a 35 yr old non-smoker and a 48 yr old one...and then yikes! All change. A sudden heading downhill at the menopause. Wrinkles, jowls, empathy lines that appear to be scored into the brow (yes, we have now started talking about me...)

Sun exposure hastens collagen's demise so wear sun hats, SPF, long sleeves, etc. You all know the drill. Our local dermatologist is 'lily white of hue' and can barely make eye contact with me as she's so worried about my sun damaged skin. I'm definitely more Californian sultana but hey ho, I try hard to cover up as much as possible now; there is an element of 'horse and stable' about it all though.

Smoking also reduces collagen production...so best to give up if you value your ability to look younger for longer (and wish to live for longer in better health of course...but let's not get into a give up smoking chat here!)

A positive addition could be phytoestrogens which I mention in the Gut chapter. These are found in plants and appear to act like oestrogens in the body. They seem to work preferentially on the oestrogen receptors within the skin (the ERbeta receptors) and one study found that they improved skin elasticity and reduced the depth of wrinkles.

Phytoestrogens are found in soybeans and other foods like grapes.

Some of the studies involve using topical oestrogen...there was one in men and women using topical oestrogen on the skin of the buttocks which did show an increase in collagen but others with no evidence of change. I'm going to have to read a bit more about this before I start crushing my oestrogen pessaries into a face mask, but I'll let you know - another thing for me to come back to you about. PS I was joking about the pessaries bit...it's a bit tricky writing stuff in a book as you're never sure who's going to take what seriously.

Hair

OK, on to hair...it sort of made sense to me to place this alongside skin, probably because dermatologists look after both things.

This is another of those mean spirited bits of the menopause; you might well be noticing more hairs on your chin and moustache area but also getting thinner hair on your scalp.

I am turning into one of those scary old aunties determined to terrify all visiting children by scooping them up into a whiskery embrace. The truly grim bit about the hairs on your chin is they're growing just when your near vision is failing so sometimes you're blithely unaware. The number of times I've found a hair 'inches' long that I've managed to miss (and all my friends and partner have obviously pretended not to notice) is too many to count.

My friends and I have a 'coma club'. The premise is that if you're in a coma, your female pals will visit regularly to de-hair you and dye your roots so that you can wake up (fingers crossed) without a full beard, etc. We are also under strict rules to point out errant lengthy whiskers...

Anyway, back to the hair on your head. You probably know this already but I'll pop it down anyway. Hair grows in three stages - a growing stage (anagen), a resting stage (catagen) and a resting then falling out stage (telogen).

Again the work is comparing women on HRT vs those who aren't. Oestrogen appears to allow hair to spend more time in the growing stage and less in the falling out stage. Without oestrogen women tend to find that their hair is thinner across the scalp.

Eyes

OK nothing to do with dermatology at all.

Dry eyes

This is felt as stinging, burning, dryness (I know that seems a stupid thing to say, but sometimes that's just how they feel - like you want to blink them a hundred times to lubricate them).

Some people describe it as feeling that they've something in their eyes, and others truly fight to get them open in the morning. Again this is not just a female thing, men and women both suffer from dry eyes.

The tear duct produces the watery part of tears and the meibomian glands produce the oily part...both are affected by oestrogen and testosterone. Reduced function of the meibomian glands appears to have the biggest influence on dry eyes problems and slightly surprisingly this is related to the dropping level of testosterone rather than oestrogen.

It's worth seeking out the usual dry eyes advice to try and help with the symptoms from this as they are difficult to live with (I've put a link in the resource sheet for my go-to leaflet).

There is an auto-immune condition called Sjogren's which is associated with dry eyes and dry mouth; if you feel that what you're getting is beyond what your pals are, then check in to make sure that this isn't the cause.

Which brings us to:

Mouth

So guess what? Yes, you guessed it, there are oestrogen receptors in the mucosal lining of the mouth and also the salivary glands. What does this mean in terms of changes at the time of the menopause?

The reported symptoms are dry mouth and burning tongue. Less saliva means that the health of the mouth reduces too leading to an increased risk of infection.

Worth having a chat with your dentist for advice on this but from what I can see - keeping well hydrated, chewing gum and sucking on ice cubes regularly can all help alleviate the symptoms.

Weight *is* a menopause issue

Let's talk about weight. This is a menopause issue and forgive me, I'm probably going to sound a bit evangelical about it.

Ageing is associated with weight gain, we know this for men and women; as we age our metabolic rate reduces and therefore we need fewer calories to do the same job.

Also a lot of us are probably slowing down a bit exercise wise (some friends have found time to restart old sporting hobbies as their children have grown but I suspect they are the minority.) Certainly perimenopausal fatigue is not conducive to much more than wanting to curl up on the couch, box of Dairy Milk in hand, with lifting the remote-control qualifying as the day's exercise.

The big change for women is that loss of oestrogen can translate, for some, into a change of shape - one day you're worrying about the size of your arse, and the next minute you have a belly on you...and often, what luck, you get to keep the arse too.

75

This is not just your regular post-baby or 'I've gained a bit of weight' tummy, you're starting to look as if you could eclipse the sun if you turned sideways; and it seems to be coming on no matter how hard you work to stop it.

It's one of those gradual changes that doesn't feel gradual - you're looking at a photo from a year before and think 'hmm, why haven't I worn those trousers in a while?', you look them out and can no longer make the buttons meet across the middle.

My subcutaneous fat (the fat layer under the skin) increased - let me tell you, doing downward dog wearing shorts was a real turning point for me, my thighs looked like a blockbuster written in Braille, dimples and bumps everywhere. Much more importantly though, for reasons I'm coming to, my central fat increased as well.

Try as I would, I couldn't seem to lose this weight. I exercised hard, I reduced my calories...two tried and tested methods that work for me when I put my mind to it...but no change, if anything it was creeping up. I went through a 'who cares' stage which was fine until I started to feel a bit short of breath when I sat down and realised that it was my abdomen pressing up on my lungs...so out came the research.

So what's happening?

This is one of those 'skip ahead to the solution if you're not keen on the background' stages.

As mentioned oestrogen generally causes women to put on weight in the 'gynoid' manner - hips and thighs. Loss of oestrogen causes us to start laying fat down in the 'android' manner - i.e. visceral fat (which surrounds the organs) and shows itself as central weight gain.

This is quite a different prospect than simply being overweight - this central weight gain is associated with a number of metabolic changes which in turn put us more at risk of diabetes, heart disease and cancer. It also means that it is difficult to lose weight because your body is now working really hard to keep hold of it and making more and more because of the disordered pathways.

The big metabolic change, which you've probably heard about, is something called insulin resistance.

Insulin is a chemical messenger; it's produced by the pancreas and it allows the cells of the body to use glucose from our diet for energy. When we eat something sugary, or something that breaks down into glucose, the pancreas responds by sending insulin into the bloodstream.

Once there, insulin acts like a genial host, unlocking the door to allow glucose to move into the cells. Here it can be used immediately or it can be stored for times that we need energy but might not have food. This storage occurs either in muscle, the liver or fat cells.

When we have used up the sugar in our blood (the immediate form of energy), we then look to our muscles to release stored energy and thereafter (and this is where it gets interesting) we start burning those fat cells to release sugar. This is the holy grail of weight loss, getting at those fat cells. You can see that if your blood is offering up a constant source of blood sugar, then you're not going to make it to fat burning.

So what's happening with insulin resistance?

For complex reasons (if you see the word complex, recognise that it made my brain quiver) the muscle cells can become resistant to insulin - i.e. the cell no longer allows insulin to open that doorway to let sugar in.

Therefore the blood sugar can't leave the bloodstream and enter the muscles as easily as it did before. The body recognises that the blood sugar isn't coming down, so it releases more insulin...and now you have two problems - high blood insulin and potentially high blood sugar.

Now that the insulin isn't working well at muscle level, it turns to the next point on its task list - the liver. Here it converts the circulating sugars into fat and this in turn can lead to a fatty liver (something that in a subgroup of people can lead to cirrhosis and liver failure over time).

Alongside insulin is converting more of your sugar into fat cells and these tend to be predominantly in the central area around the organs (i.e. not good fat; there is good fat, it's just that this isn't it). This fat, the visceral fat, releases inflammatory markers which in turn lead to greater insulin resistance and round and round the circle we go.

I have totally oversimplified this and undoubtedly physiologists will be shaking their heads sadly at me - I have put a book recommendation in the resource sheet which deals with insulin resistance. I had to read some of the research papers a few times before I got my foggy brain to absorb the information.

So, the perimenopause hits and we start getting this central weight gain, that in turn causes insulin resistance which in turn causes a high level of circulating insulin. This excess insulin has far reaching consequences, not just those listed above; it can affect the way your appetite works (it makes you want to reach for the quick-to-use calories = refined carbohydrates), it can influence inflammatory pathways which in turn can lead to some cancers, it can change the ratio of your good to your bad cholesterol which in turn can lead to heart disease.

In addition to all of this, lack of sleep is conspiring against you by making you think you need to eat more (we'll come to this later)...seriously you couldn't make it up; it's like your body suddenly becomes a glucose-craving, fat-creating monster.

What to do?!

Even when you're making your best effort to lose weight, this sometimes isn't enough. What you're eating becomes as important as how much you're eating, and the type of exercise you do can also have an impact.

Perimenopausal women have to start looking at nutrition in a slightly different way. Quite simply, it's worth acting as if someone just told you that you've got diabetes, and believe you me, insulin resistance is essentially a pathway to diabetes if left to its own devices.

Nutrition

Reduce sugar. If we think of ourselves as being diabetic, what's the first thing that comes to mind? Sugar. So this is a good place to start.

Essentially not all calories are born equal, your body treats your sugar calorie differently to your protein calorie. This is where the simple 'calories in/calories out' advice starts to fall down. I could take my daily calorie intake as chocolate, or I could take it as salad and although I'm eating 2000 calories each day, my body will punish me for the chocolate and be significantly more gracious about the salad.

Sugar is not just sugar as we think of it - the white stuff in the bowl or that you add to your baking. Refined carbohydrates are quickly converted into glucose in the body, so are the same as sugar hits. Carbohydrates which are broken down slowly supply a more steady release of glucose.

This is where all the Glycaemic Index information comes into its own, a low GI food is one that releases glucose gradually into the bloodstream e.g. oatbran, whereas a high GI one goes full impact, high sugar hit e.g. white pasta. You can see that high GI = bad, low GI = good.

If you do want to start losing weight by reducing your sugar intake then a good rule of thumb is to check the side of the packet and see what the sugar content per 100g is and aim for 4 and fewer. Now, I don't do this, my favourite yoghurt is 4.7g/100g and my favourite frozen berries are a bit more, so when I'm really paying attention to this and want to shift some kilos, I set my marker a bit higher...5/100g. I don't believe in making something unachievable so I have to be honest with myself...I don't have the world's best will power and I do love food.

That said, it really is an eye opener when you start looking at sugar content. The bakers amongst you know that homemade Victoria Sponge is nearly a third sugar and when you buy a processed cake, it's likely the sugar content is even higher. A rather innocuous sounding 'luxury fruit toast' from a high street cafe has 39 g sugar per 100g. Sugar also sneaks into places you don't expect to see it, like processed sauces and pizzas.

There's nothing I'm telling you here that you don't know already, but sugar has become something more of a villain now you're perimenopausal so it bears repeating.

In addition to that consider changing your nutrition in line, as much as possible, with the Mediterranean diet. Doctors everywhere, myself included, love the Mediterranean diet and it's an easy one to follow as a lifestyle choice, alongside the above. It's all about 'brown' carbs (which sadly doesn't mean chocolate but does mean wild rice, wholewheat pasta...), lots of veggies and pulses e.g. chickpeas, lentils, etc. Olive oil, nuts, occasional glass of red wine...and so on. Looks pretty palatable when it's written down like that.

I have to remind myself though that there can be too much of a good thing - eating a handful of nuts a day is great, eating twenty-seven handfuls, not so much...the calories in/calories out still counts in that circumstance!

Fasting

One of the things that helped me lose my gradually gained kilos, was intermittent fasting and the science supports this, as it particularly tackles insulin resistance and that central weight gain.

I started with the 5:2, i.e. eating 800 calories for two days out of seven and then when I'd lost my weight, I reduced to one day per week to maintain the loss...and then I fell off the wagon. I'm not sure why but I did and my weight is starting to go up and I'm in a slightly devil-may-care mood of waiting until the Spring to try and change this! I am a sublime case of 'do as I say, but not as I do'.

The other good way to fast is to have a 16 hour break from food, this really means just missing a meal a day and you can do this every day or maybe, particularly if you're perimenopausal, take one day off a week.

Fat burning starts at 12 hours of fasting, so you can see that any amount that you can extend that time by will be beneficial. The fasted period gives your liver time to concentrate on fulfilling its other roles and not just spend its time processing calories.

The other good news is that the central weight is the bit that seems to disappear first. (Woo hoo!)

You have to find what works for you. There are plenty of good nutritional pathways to follow and what works for me won't necessarily work for you, but insulin resistance is a key here and so choose something that acknowledges that change that you're undergoing.

And whilst it is easy to lose heart, *any* weight loss will have an impact on that visceral fat so even if you're not changing shape quickly, you will still be making a difference.

Personally, when it comes to lifestyle change, I have to employ the 80:20 principle (although I'm not sure what the real 80:20 principle means but I'm using it for my own ends) where I try to be good for 80% of the time and don't beat myself up for that 20% when I run free. However if you're not losing weight, then you might need to be kinder to yourself and go for the full 100%, follow the rules with whatever regime you choose until that weight has gone and only then allow a bit of slack...by which time, you probably won't want to slack anyway as you'll be feeling more energetic and not craving sugar.

I hadn't planned to write this much as there are lots of people out there who've written well on this and I'd recommend that you seek them out. I've put some recommendations in the resource sheet at the end.

<u>Exercise</u>

Exercise of any sort helps reduce insulin resistance. It does this by driving sugar into the muscles via a different doorway than the one that needs insulin as the key. So walking, yoga, climbing, running, etc. will all help.

Don't jump straight into a full-on exercise programme if you're not exercising at all. I heard a doctor the other day talking about a phased return and I liked his idea.

If you're carrying a lot of weight, then use diet to try and reduce this by a bit first of all. Then start doing something three times per week, a gentle walk or swim. Add some stretching, then increase to something gentle five times a week, add some weight training and then increase intensity from there.

Weight training is good as you're creating more muscle which will scoop up more of that sugar which in turn leads to less insulin production and we start closing down that vicious cycle once and for all.

If you want to really science it out, then high intensity interval training (HIIT) appears to selectively increase the burning of the central fat and really supports the use of the alternate gateway for pushing glucose into the muscles, so you get a lot of benefit from your single programme.

Again, this is the bit that made the difference for me. If I fast without doing HIIT then I don't lose as much weight, mix the two together and it is like magic.

There's a 7 minute exercise programme developed by the American College of Sports Medicine, I love the Pop Sugar version on YouTube as she's a sweetie and pretends that it's hurting when it obviously isn't but it makes you feel better. I love psychology that I can see through but still works!

Of course as a yoga teacher, I'm all about yoga as an exercise solution with benefits. It helps with muscle building, fat burning and also, as a by-product, brings calm, balance and flexibility...what's not to love?

Again, it's a case of finding what works for you and remembering every little bit makes a difference.

Microbiome

There's a lot of work coming out about how the gut microbiome (the bacteria in the gut) can influence everything from weight gain and insulin resistance to mood and more and I'll talk a bit more about this in the gut chapter.

So whilst I didn't really want to make the menopause about weight. I think for me, it is an important opportunity to share the chance of improving your health despite the fact that your body appears to be actively working against you.

Skinny looking people with normal BMI (body mass index) can still have insulin resistance and visceral fat. How do you know?

We can measure waist:hip ratios (your waist measurement divided by your hip measurement) to assess visceral fat. In women, you want your Waist to Hip Ratio to be less than 0.85. Another quick check is to see if your waist is bigger than 80cms, if it is then you probably want to consider making some changes.

One study I read showed that waist: height ratio corresponded most closely with the amount of visceral fat seen on a specialised scanner. You divide your waist measurement by your height and you're aiming to be in >35 and <49.

As a doctor, I know that weight is a sensitive issue, people get really upset when doctors talk to them about their weight. Whilst we can live without cigarettes, we actually do need to carry on eating to survive so it's really difficult to find a path through this. Food sets off signals in the brain that can comfort us, thus it's not surprising that it's difficult to walk away from something that essentially is making us feel better and that we need to live.

That said, obesity (i.e. BMI over 30) is the second biggest preventable cause of cancer. Second to smoking. I'm not sure that's something a lot of people know. At least 1 in 20 cancers have been caused by excess weight. Don't get me wrong, not every obese person will get cancer, but the longer a person is overweight for and also the higher their weight is, the more likely they will be to get cancer.

Risk Factors by Number of **Preventable** Cases, UK, Persons, 2015 (Cancer Research UK) (Cited 2021)

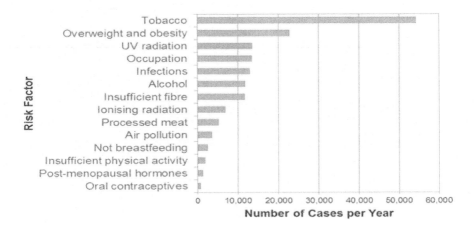

Insulin resistance is associated with an increased risk of heart disease, even if you don't go on to develop diabetes, and heart disease remains the number one cause of death globally according to the World Health Organisation (WHO), and is the leading cause of death for women in the Western world.

We generally think of weight as being a cosmetic issue, the 'does my bum look big in this?' but it's so much more for some of us.

It is intricately caught up in our self-esteem. Whilst we wouldn't think twice about telling one of our mates to give up smoking, it wouldn't cross our minds to advise that they lose weight. People write to complain when their doctors have told them to lose weight; now, don't get me wrong, there are good ways to discuss weight and bad, some doctors definitely fall at the ultra practical/tough talking end of the spectrum when it comes to having this discussion which might not be the right way in for some people.

The thing is we often don't notice that we've gained weight. Currently I'm writing this in Lockdown V3 and I've spent my non-working hours in yoga pants, and my working ones in scrubs or an old, large pair of trousers that I can wash on 60 degrees. I popped a pair of jeans on last weekend to go walking and yikes! they pinch...actually that's an understatement, they cause my belly to rise into my rib cage and make sitting difficult. I need to do something now.

As a doctor, I've started normalising the size of people who see me in clinic and when I put them on the scales or check their waist circumference, I'm as much surprised that they're 'obese' as they are.

93

So if you're looking to doctors to tell you you're overweight and we haven't, that doesn't mean you aren't!

I'm always interested in what the trigger has been for someone when they do lose weight and one lady shared that when she was seen for her check up, following her second baby, the doctor (a practical, say it like it is, female), told her in no uncertain terms that she was obese and that she needed to lose weight.

She went home and cried, and then felt really angry and thought about writing a letter of complaint; however a few days passed and she decided that she'd 'show that doctor' and did just that.

She lost 31 kilos / 5 stone and felt one thousand times better for it.

In retrospect she realises that the doctor's recommendation was a gift; this was not a change she would have made herself. When she looked in the mirror, she saw that she'd gained a bit of weight but had no idea how much and it's only now looking back at photos that she realised just how much extra weight she was carrying.

A long story to demonstrate that we normalise our own weight over time and it might need an outside party, mate/mother/doctor, to let us know that we've gained some and the time has come to lose it...a gift to improve life, not a criticism.

What else? I think that's probably it for weight for now. I'm hoping you'll see that it *is* harder to lose weight now, your body is fighting hard to stop you but it is possible to do and there is an enormous benefit to doing so.

To bleed or not to bleed

So let's move to something which you have no control over and is going to do exactly whatever it fancies, when it fancies...your bleed pattern.

(Slight caveat here: there is work coming through on the microbiome which suggests we may have the opportunity to exert a small influence on this too, another of those 'watch this space' moments that I'll update on IG).

There are three main ways the bleeding pattern can change at the perimenopause.

You can simply stop having periods...this is what happened to me. (That's not quite true, I broke my ankle about nine months after I'd had what I'd thought was my last period, and then had a bleed. I mention this because it demonstrates how interconnected our hormones are and how this completely non-gynae but physiologically stressful event led to a short-lived restart of my cycle.

Of course, at the time I didn't wow in the beauty of the hormones, I was non-weight bearing and now also had a period...I was grumpy as hell).

The cycle can become shorter, and then over time longer gaps may fall between the periods until they stop completely.

Or, and this is the grim one, the cycle goes all over the shop - two to three months without, then bleeding non stop for weeks on end.

This last one involves anovulatory cycles - i.e. cycles in which ovulation hasn't occurred.

To get your head around what's happening it is helpful to know what's happening in the usual cycle with the womb lining.

For the first part of the cycle, oestrogen is building up the lining of the womb, then, at ovulation, progesterone is produced and this has a direct effect on stabilising and thickening the lining of the womb, readying it to welcome a fertilised egg. When fertilisation doesn't occur both oestrogen and progesterone levels drop and the lining of the womb is shed.

If ovulation doesn't occur, which happens more frequently as the ovary ages, then oestrogen just continues to act on the lining building it up and there isn't a clear signal for when to bleed, so instead there can be spotting, clotting and heavy bleeding seemingly whenever the womb fancies.

Doctors are keen to hear about and will likely investigate any changes from your normal bleeding pattern, particularly prolonged, unstructured bleeding episodes. Other symptoms of concern are bleeding between the periods or bleeding after sex, new pain and new discharge. Long story short, check in to make sure that what's happening is perimenopause and nothing more.

This really causes much more heartache that this few line summary seems to imply. It doesn't seem fair really; however doctors have a bunch of treatments they can offer (after investigating fully) so seek them out rather than putting up with this.

Of course, lots of women, as a result of their contraceptive choice, don't have periods at all during their forties. The progesterone only pill and the intrauterine system (IUS) often stop the monthly bleed; this can make it difficult to know if you're menopausal or not and I cover this further in the contraception chapter.

Genitourinary syndrome of the menopause anyone?!

Yup, I didn't make that title up, this is the new moniker for the changes in the lower urinary tract, vagina and vulva with peri and postmenopause. To be fair, we used to refer to the changes as atrophic vaginitis (thin inflamed vagina) and urogenital atrophy, so let's be honest, it's a bit better than those. I think we can safely say that doctors won't be winning any naming competitions any time soon though.

I have loved the names that I've heard over the years for the vaginal and external genital area. 'Down below', 'front bottom', 'mini', 'miffin', 'muffin' (not sure why the m's get such a look in) and so the list goes on.

For the purposes of this chapter we're going to be talking about the genito-urinary system: 'genito' referring to all things gynae: womb, ovaries, cervix, vagina and the external genitalia - the vulva (the large and small lips outside the vagina) and the clitorus. The 'urinary' in this instance is referring to the bladder and the exit from the bladder to the outside- the urethra (which appears smack bang in the middle of the external genitalia).

I won't be overdoing it when I speak of this as a 'drying up' from the inside out...OK, I might be a bit. The tissues of these areas are thinning, they're more fragile, and less elastic, and also the mucus production is less efficient.

There is a triangular area in the bladder that loves oestrogen too and without it this area thins and becomes more fragile.

The whole look of the vulva and clitoral hood may change - literally shrinking away, and this leads to exposure of the hidden more sensitive tissues.

Back in the day, we used to laugh jokingly about a period of sexual abstinence leading to a sealing up from underuse...well, joke no more. This menopausal change can lead to a shortening of the vagina, tightening of the vaginal entrance and more!

As with all the menopause symptoms, not everyone gets this...I think of menopause symptoms as a sort of reverse smorgasbord where you don't get to choose what you eat but you get served by someone who is having a bad day. With this particular set of symptoms you have to imagine that you've really, really offended the grumpiest waiter/waitress you've ever encountered, *and* they've decided you're not going to tip.

The most recent studies show that 50% of women over the age of 50 suffer from symptoms; and far more pertinent, of those 50% only 10% seek help.

Wow, wow, wow. That means in a crew of 100 women, 50 have vaginal symptoms that are probably wiping their sex lives out and making them wriggle whilst trying to sit still, and yet only 5 of them are seeking help. Sorry, I know you know maths but it felt important to run those numbers in a different way.

And what about sex drive?

As we all know sexual desire is a complex mix of psychological and physical factors.

There are lots of good reasons why your sex drive might be falling after the age of 40 - you're knackered as you're sleeping badly, your self esteem has hit rock bottom, you generally feel a bit low, your family are scooping up all of your energy and maybe you spend more time thinking about your partner's annoying habits than you do their endearing ones.

It may, or may not, be reassuring to hear that the menopause plays a direct part in this too.

Your ovaries and your adrenal glands create your sex hormones, the big hitters that we've talked a lot about - oestrogen and progesterone- but also testosterone and androstenedione. It's not fully understood how but there is a definite interplay between these, directly influencing your libido (your desire to have sex).

If you think back to your usual period cycle, you probably realised that there were times that you were super up for sex and other times in the cycle when chocolate felt like the best way to push up your feel good chemicals.

Some of this cyclical change in sex drive is thought to be part of evolution, it makes sense for you to be on your game at ovulation, thereby giving that egg its best chance at being fertilised. After the menopause there isn't an egg to be fertilised so that evolutionary need has passed.

It isn't really clear how much each hormone impacts on libido. It was thought that testosterone might be a strong player. It falls at the time of the menopause but is still present (I am so putting the hairs on my chin down to this); but there doesn't seem to be significant evidence for it supporting libido any more than the others. However, in research when women were given testosterone gel to treat low sex drive there seemed to be some benefit although the studies are small and short-lived.

So the impulse to have sex is affected; and in addition to this, there are these very real physical changes to the vaginal and vulval tissues that are playing a profound part too.

So let's walk through it and if you think you have these symptoms, and this is the only time I'm going to be directive in this book, please speak to a doctor, nurse, pharmacist or your healthcare provider of choice about it. This is one symptom of the menopause that doesn't get better with time - flushes will pass, palpitations will pass but *this*, if you have it, will just continue.

How does this feel to begin with?

Dryness is the first symptom women tend to present with, then itching, a constant feeling of the area being irritable. Soreness, not just during sex, but generally. Essentially a persistent low grade discomfort.

By not creating enough mucus during sex to lubricate the wheels, sex becomes painful. The brain doesn't need to feel pain too many times before it starts thinking that it would be better avoiding that stressor (hence the fact that we don't spend our days hitting our thumb with a hammer) so at the next sexual encounter, there might be a fear, even at subconscious level, which leads to spasm (vaginismus) = more pain.

The change in the vaginal mucus also leads to a change in acidity - it becomes less acid and this can lead to an increase in discharge and a change in the natural bacterial protection (the vaginal microbiome). There may be more thrush or bacterial vaginosis infections.

In addition to the above, the fragility in the bladder and the bladder exit can lead to repeated urine infections. It can also lead to passing urine more often, including getting up more often at night (like you needed your sleep any more disturbed).

You may develop urge incontinence - this is when from the moment you realise you need the loo, you have to run like billy-o to ensure you get there before wetting yourself.

The tissues holding the womb and bladder up become thinner and less strong too and prolapse of the vaginal walls can occur. Stress incontinence is when you laugh or sneeze and a small/large amount of urine pops out, that's related to the pelvic floor changing too. Traditionally that's been associated with large pregnancies and difficult deliveries but this happens to women who haven't had children and those who delivered by caesarean.

What to do?!

- Avoid bubble baths, perfumed products, feminine hygiene sprays (I have no idea what these are), etc.

- Ideally try not to wear pads - particularly not ones with perfumes.

- Pat yourself dry after showering (one of my patients found using a hairdryer best).

- Pee after sex (no newbie but worth remembering).

Pelvic floor muscle exercises

By strengthening this area you reduce the risk of stress incontinence and likely byproduct, improve sexual pleasure too.

I can't emphasise enough how important this is.

So many women suffer in silence and the only people who are benefiting from that seem to be the pad manufacturers.

If you have incontinence or a prolapse then doing your pelvic floor exercises can be really successful.

A Cochrane review of pelvic floor exercises for stress incontinence (the cough/laugh one) showed women were 8 x more likely to be cured and 17 x more likely to say that they'd improved after doing them.

The secret of success is a four month course - 10 slow 10 second holds, followed by 50 short holds...repeated three times a day.

I've attached a link for Kegel exercises. There is a squeezy app which reminds you to get pulsing...because let's be honest, we all start out motivated and after about a day or two, we've fallen by the wayside.

There are biofeedback devices you can buy that will let you know how well you're doing these exercises and also, as everything is linked to your phone now, send you reminders that you should be squeezing.

If you're struggling, you've done all the above or simply can't seem to work out how to, then please refer yourself to see a gynae physiotherapist who can help with this. Most of these accept self referrals now or you can access through your doctor's surgery.

Any exercise that improves your pelvic floor e.g. Pilates and yoga will be beneficial but I'd really recommend doing the exercise programme above...even if you don't yet have a problem.

So no surprises that I've managed to find a way to pop yoga on to the list of treatments!

There was a study in the Journal of Sexual Medicine that looked at women of all ages and their sexual function. 75% felt their sex lives did improve at the end of a 12 week course of daily yoga practice.

This may be related to the improvement in the pelvic floor - mula bandha is a lock that we employ during some yoga poses and breathing exercises, and it is essentially strengthening the pelvic floor.

However, as much as I like to fit yoga into all the menopause solutions, the study didn't compare with women who weren't doing yoga so it's tricky to take much from this study. If they'd asked women to climb two flights of stairs every day for twelve weeks, chances are they'd have got similar results - exercise generally makes us feel better, happier, lighter and more energetic.

I think what this study shows is that yoga makes women feel better generally and as a result they enjoy sex more.

And, in the spirit of 'if you don't use it, you lose it', even if you're not in a relationship, remaining active is a good way to keep the vaginal tissue more elastic - whilst a patient of mine said that '...she can't unsee...' some of the devices on the sex shop website, she does appreciate the fact that she could order and have her vibrator delivered in a nice brown paper package, without having to endure the postie giving her a knowing look.

What else?

Well, on a day-to-day/as needed basis, you can use water-based lubricants. They're very much in the here and now, you use them for comfort and at the time of sex. You have to take a bit of care as some of these can affect how well condoms work (more about condoms in the next chapter).

There are also vaginal moisturizers. Now these are different from lubricants because you use them every two or three days and they increase the moisture by working directly on the vaginal cells increasing their hydration. Much more useful in terms of spontaneity!

It is recommended to do a patch test on the skin before using any of these products vaginally. Check to see how the skin is after 24hrs and no irritation and redness should be reassuring.

Try to ensure that there are as few additives as possible...perfumes still seem to make their way into these products which feels counterintuitive, but I guess manufacturers like to make things smell nice. Some of the products contain parabens and glycols which may have a negative effect on the vaginal biome (the good bacteria) too.

The pre-menopausal vaginal pH is slightly acidic - water is 7.0 on the pH scale, anything acidic has a pH below 7 and alkaline has a pH above 7. Therefore you'd be best to choose something with a similar pH (3.8 - 4.5) as this is the level that the good bacteria are used to flourishing in.

There needs to be osmolar balance. If the lubricant has a stronger osmolality than the vaginal cell it will draw water out of the cell, if it's too weak then too much water might end up in the vaginal cell. There is a Goldilocks 'just right' amount of push and pull which leaves the cell hydrated but not damaged.

So how are you supposed to know what to buy?! The list above could have you standing in the pharmacy aisle for hours as you check the pH and the products, etc. and throw in the fact that you've forgotten your glasses and can't read the small print...where on earth do you start?

I've attached a link to the paper that investigated this really thoroughly and midway through this there is a table that shows which ones had good pH and better osmolality. Now bear in mind that this study was done in 2015 so things may have changed but it's a good place to start.

Then we come to what you can get on prescription.

Topical oestrogen i.e. in a form that acts locally on the vaginal tissues, can also be offered on prescription. Generally this can be used as a ring inserted into the vagina, creams or pessaries (tablets you pop inside the vagina).

Doctors offer this for all the symptoms listed above; because it is only working locally, it is often available even for women who aren't allowed to have hormone replacement therapy. This is going to be part of the discussion that you have with your doctor/nurse if you decide to speak with them.

The pessaries can be something of an eco nightmare as some come with a disposable plastic applicator for each dose, but drug companies are waking up to waste so if you do decide to choose this route then I reckon you can find a pathway through to the least impactful (is that a word?) and word on the street is that they're moving to cardboard.

There are a couple of new products on the market too, they've not made it to a lot of guidelines yet. One, DHEA (dehydroepiandrosterone) is used locally as a pessary and converts to oestrogen, it's licensed for moderate or severe symptoms. The other is a tablet to swallow, which is called ospemifene. This has an 'oestrogenic' effect on the vaginal cells. I suspect both will remain in the territory of menopause specialists and gynaecologists for some time to come and certainly haven't made it to the UK's guidelines yet, but it's good to see new products coming through.

And then, LASER! Yes, you heard me right, the Buzz Lightyear treatment. Am I the only one who thinks of Buzz when laser is mentioned? I'm worrying that I might have some deep-seated Toy Story stuff going on.

Until I started looking into the menopause I had not heard of this at all but when I did read about it, it made perfect sense. Now don't get too excited, in a lot of countries this is still only available in research studies or privately. It works on the same principle as the laser used on the face to reduce wrinkles by improving the amount of collagen and elastin in the skin.

So there you go, vaginal laser treatment, coming to a cover of Hello magazine soon.

Contraception and sexual health

Contraception - YOU STILL NEED IT!

So that's my main message. Ooh and CONDOMS - PLEASE STILL USE THEM if you're dating...more on that in a bit.

The stopping of periods doesn't mean that you are no longer fertile. This is a common misconception and why boring chapter number one with all its dates in the diary is so important.

I have seen a number of women in their late forties surprised to find themselves pregnant. I thank that little guardian doctor angel that sits on my shoulder, which makes me ask some women to do a pregnancy test when I don't remember to do this for everyone.

Many of the contraception choices allow women to stop having periods - the IUS (a coil with progesterone) and also the progesterone only pill, implant and injection. Therefore many women can be unsure when they're going through their menopause as they don't have that last period date - they simply don't have any periods at all. The risk with this is that some stop their contraception and think they can run free without really being sure if they're menopausal or not.

Just last week when I asked a 49 yr old woman what she was using for contraception, she told me that she wasn't using anything...and yes, she was still sexually active. She'd had her IUS taken out the previous year having not had a bleed for eight years whilst on it (the no bleed is a direct effect of the hormone in the coil). She assumed that she didn't need to use anything else thereafter. Pregnancy test alert! She was presenting with bloating and nausea - lots of things can cause this, but in an un-contracepted woman pregnancy test is the first investigation, only then followed by bloods. Cue lots of squealing.

Great, we've established that we do still need to use contraception but for how long?

118

If you go through your menopause pre-50, the advice is contraception for two years after the last period. And if you go through your menopause post 50 then the recommendation is for one year after your last period.

I've written that down in the resource sheet so you don't have to try and remember where in the book to find this.

Obviously you might be like me and not really remember when your last period was. I'd simply take the date that you realise that you've been period free and just add the years to that...there is a blood test but who wants a blood test if they don't need one and it's a way to avoid the eye-roll of the tired physician who wonders how flaky you can be not to remember when your last period was (as flaky as me, it would seem!)

If you're on the IUS or progesterone only pill, then chances are you may not be having periods and haven't for some years. It's recommended now that if you're over 50 you can have an FSH test and if it's raised then you add one year of contraception. If you're under 50 the recommendation is that you continue taking contraception and only have a check > 50 yrs.

Unfortunately if you're on the combined pill, HRT or injection, this won't work as the hormones in these have a direct effect on the FSH level. (With the injection in fact, you can have the blood test just before your injection is due as the level of hormone will be quite low by then).

The combined pill isn't prescribed after the age of 50, so you could move to the progesterone only pill or IUS at this stage...this is certainly recommended rather than the usual advice of stopping the pill for six weeks before doing the blood tests...therein all manner of risk lies!

If you don't know when your menopause was then it's recommended that you use contraception until you're 55 yrs old.

Whilst these are the just-updated rules, they certainly may change so it's a good one to double check when the time comes.

I'm not going to get into different types of contraception here but I certainly have my favourites and you'll find that loads of female doctors over 40 have the IUS; it offers lighter bleeds at a time your bleed pattern is worsening, it provides sterling levels of contraception and it can be used as the progesterone bit of your HRT if you decide to go that route. Come find me to talk this through more.

And now on to sexual health…

The one massive positive of moving beyond the menopause is the opportunity to celebrate the freedom of no periods and, at some stage, you'd think, no contraception.

However I'm going to caveat that big time. Sexual transmitted infections (STIs) don't have feelings, they don't recognise all the rest of the hell you're going through and think 'do you know what, let's let her be, she's embracing her new found freedom and she deserves that.' If you're embracing your Tinder spirit, condoms are still the only way to avoid HIV, chlamydia, gonorrhoea and all the other gloriously named infections out there.

In Britain, the most recent Natsal study (the National Survey of Sexual Attitudes and Lifestyles) showed a 140% increase in numbers of women over 50 visiting their local sexual health clinic from the previous study (2011 vs 2013). Age UK supported a study recently that was published in the Student BMJ that revealed a doubling of STIs in the 50-90 yr old population.

Women tend to get worried about seeking out their doctor or nurse to discuss their sexual health. They often feel they're going to be judged in some way (you're not, by the way, generally we're just congratulatory with a small dose of big sister thrown in to make sure you're staying safe). New discharge, lower abdominal pain, urine infection after urine infection - these could all be related to STIs so give us the chance to support you here and come find us.

Since Covid, many of the sexual health clinics offer remote testing - how brilliant is that?! You'll receive a kit through the post (brown paper packaging of course) and you can be tested from the comfort of your own home. All clear but still symptoms, then book to see your doctor.

The vaginal microbiome - the bacteria that naturally reside in the vagina to keep it healthy - changes after the menopause and this increases the opportunity for bacterial vaginosis and thrush infections. These aren't sexually transmitted but they do have an impact in terms of discomfort, itching and increased vaginal discharge...BV can bring an odour too - such delight.

So again, condoms for preventing HIV and the rest (that Age UK study showed that the greatest increase in STIs is in the 50 - 59 male group...which might, or might not, be your perfect pick on that dating app.)

Gut changes and the microbiome

OK, this is where my inner doctor gets properly overexcited. This is a whole new area of medicine for me - we weren't taught anything about the microbiome in medical school because it truly wasn't a thing back then. In fact, I don't remember being taught anything about the menopause either but that's a different story. If you're listening to this on audio, you may want to slow me down...

So let's lead out with the gut symptoms that women may see at the time of the menopause, I will preface this by saying that any change in your toileting habit, or new 'abdominal' symptoms e.g bloating, indigestion, pain, blood seen, etc. benefit from a check-in with your doctor. You're at an age where other problems would need to be excluded before we would consider any change to be menopause related.

The main change seen for some is constipation - usual habit is having your bowels open once to twice daily and if you're falling beneath this threshold then that's going to start leading to problems with tummy pain, bloating later in the day, straining and occasionally loose motions as the softer stool bypasses the obstructing hard stool. Some women find that they get more indigestion symptoms and others develop acid reflux.

So why would oestrogen have a direct influence on this part of our body? Well, it may surprise you to hear that there are oestrogen receptors in the gut; this hormone that we've previously only really associated with our period cycle, plays a role in the health of the gut.

Oestrogen helps keep the gut healthy, ensuring the integrity of the gut wall, by keeping the cells tightly knitted together. As oestrogen drops with the perimenopause, the gut can become 'leaky'. This allows toxins that are made in the gut (endotoxins) to leak through into the bloodstream which, let's be honest, doesn't sound good. The endotoxins are called lipopolysaccharides and once in the bloodstream play a part in increasing central weight gain, cause the problems with insulin that we've already discussed.

Oestrogen also plays a part in supporting the mucus lining of the stomach, this protects the stomach against the acid that is produced there. We need this acid to kill off toxins and also to digest our food,

126

but it is strong and would damage the stomach lining without this mucus layer. Men are significantly more likely to get cancer of the stomach in their lifetime compared with women and it's wondered if this oestrogenic support of the mucus lining and the tight junctions between the cells are part of the reason for this.

Alongside this, the gut plays a part in clearing oestrogen from our bodies. Oestrogen passes to the liver where it's packaged up and sent to the gut in the bile to be sent out with usual waste. The gut has its own recycling system that can influence your oestrogen levels by causing some of your 'discarded' oestrogen to be taken back up into the bloodstream. This recycling system is called the estrobolome and is part of your microbiome...which we will come to now.

Before I explain more about the microbiome, it's useful to note here that we know oestrogen has a direct effect on the health of the microbiome, increasing its diversity i.e. the number of different strains of microbe that exist within it.

Amazing!

So what's the microbiome and what role does it play in our health and particularly our postmenopausal health?

Our body houses trillions of microbes - bacteria, fungi, viruses. The term microbiome refers to these microbes, their genes and the surrounding environment. We have these microbes on our skin, in our vagina, in our bowel and more.

How did they get there? There seems to be a bit of work to show that there may be some transfer through the placenta but the main early exposures are at birth specifically via vaginal delivery, skin to skin contact, and through the breast milk. A child born by caesarean section is found to have more hospital microbes as part of their gut bacteria until about six to nine months when the difference has disappeared.

It keeps developing and by about three years of age has hit 'adult' form.

As we grow, our microbiome is influenced by what we eat, whether we're stressed, if we've taken antibiotics, whether we exercise and a bunch of other things.

What we're after is a healthy microbiome and this means a diverse one with as many different types of bacteria as possible. There also needs to be a balance between the gut communities, if one is over-represented then it is likely that will lead to problems. There are some real stars that we should try and get more of and others that, ideally, should play less of a leading role.

There are some beautiful names. Who wouldn't want more Akkermansia muciniphila in their life? Not only does it sound gorgeous, it appears to reduce metabolic syndrome (diabetes, obesity, high blood pressure ++) and atherosclerosis (the fatty build up on the lining of arteries). What's not to love?

Whilst each of us has our very own microbiome which is as individual as our fingerprint, it has been found that the general makeup of the microbiome fits into patterns within communities.

129

I find this all really interesting as Ayurvedic medicine deals with three doshas or constitutional types, and much of its practice involves individualised nutritional care based on your predominant type. Some people are a mix of two or all three in varying levels and there is the rare person out there who is one dosha only. Research into Ayurvedic medicine is already looking at how the doshas may relate to the microbial make up.

Whilst the current advice is very general for how to support the microbiome, it won't be long before you can find out exactly what your microbiome looks like and therefore eat for it (this is already happening privately through some companies and remains research based with others e.g. ZOE). This will be important because some food choices that look healthy, e.g. broccoli, may turn out not to be for some individuals.

For now it's best to try and stick to the general rules which are, reassuringly, all the nutrition and exercise changes that we've already talked about in the previous chapter plus a few things that taste good that you can add too. I'll dip into this again at the end of this chapter to redefine in terms of the biome, but I didn't want you to start feeling overwhelmed that there was another nutrition change pending.

So why bother? Well, and here's where it becomes so interesting, the microbiome can influence many areas of the body and, for me, the most stunning of all is the brain.

In the mood chapter I allude to the fact that we can eat ourselves happy and I wasn't being glib. Our diet does have a profound effect on the microbiome and in turn on how happy or sad or anxious or worried we feel. We might think that eating ourselves happy means chocolate cake and ice cream (it's called comfort eating after all); but, as you've probably guessed, chocolate cake isn't the right foodstuff for improving your microbiome. However a good quality dark chocolate might be. Woo hoo! Take away with one hand, give with the other.

The effect of the microbiome is being explored for its impact on the mood, anxiety, autism, Alzheimer's, schizophrenia, Parkinson's and more. Did you know that 85% of our serotonin, our 'feel-good' chemical is found within the gut? I know! I did not know this, I thought that the majority of serotonin was made in the brain.

A good, diverse microbiome has been associated with less obesity, better lipid (cholesterol and triglycerides) profiles, increased insulin sensitivity, improved fertility. If your microbiome is out of kilter then it can mean that you don't lose weight, even if you seem to be trying your utmost to do so; it comes down to what you're eating and your utmost may need a nutritional tweak.

This is such a huge subject that I'm going to suggest a book or two that you might want to read if you'd like to know more; however I am going to share the general rules for keeping your biome as diverse as possible. Bear in mind that the diversity reduces as we age and as mentioned already, oestrogen has a direct effect on improving diversity and we now have significantly less of that.

The most important thing you can do is eat fibre. Why? Soluble fibre is a prebiotic i.e. it creates the right environment for the good gut bacteria to thrive.

Fibre comes in two forms - soluble and insoluble. It's the insoluble fibre that we've concentrated on historically - the bit that simply comes out the other end, it's generally cellulose and is the cell walls of the plant that can't be digested. It does provide benefit though as it provides an architecture on which to create the stool.

It's soluble fibre I'm talking about from here on though. This can't be digested in the small intestine, but when it transits to the large intestine it is welcomed by the microbiome for whom it is the equivalent of chocolate and champagne...The microbiome ferments the soluble fibre and turns it into short chain fatty acids (SCFA). These sound as though they're bad since they've got fat in the name but they are the absolute opposite of bad.

The best known is probably butyrate and this has been shown to increase insulin sensitivity. It has an effect on regulating the appetite, lowering cholesterol, boosting the immunity and reducing gut leakiness. It also selectively goes after that visceral fat, triggering the metabolism to burn these fat cells rather than sugar for energy.

You make this yourself if you supply the gut with the right nutrients. Bonus! And no extra money needing to be spent than your normal grocery shop.

So how do you get your hands on that fibre? It's found in complex carbohydrates which are your plant based foods. Guess where it isn't found...yup, sugar and processed foods. These are the ones to avoid if you're hoping to have a healthy biome.

Here's the plan:

Nutrition

Eat at least 30 different plant based foods per week - I have to admit when I first heard that my heart fell. I couldn't name 30 veggies, let alone work out if they were in my diet. Reassuringly though, plant-based means wholegrains (e.g. quinoa, rice, oats), legumes (e.g. chickpeas, lentils and beans), nuts, seeds, veggies and fruit. Phew!

Onions, leeks and garlic are good because they contain inulin which is a soluble fibre.

Anything with polyphenols is great - so peppers, tomatoes, olives, berries - the rainbow plate of food. Good news fact, polyphenols appear in red wine, chocolate and extra virgin olive oil. There are polyphenols in lots of herbs and spices. I'll put the European Journal of Clinical Nutritions 'Top 100 polyphenol containing foods' in the resource sheet.

Seeds are interesting, linseed mimics oestrogen (in a good way) when it's converted by the microbiome. You have to eat milled linseed or otherwise they simply appear unchanged at the other end. Good way to work out how fast your transit time is though.

Foods that have this mild oestrogenic effect are called phytoestrogens and you may have heard of Red Clover which is a supplement version of one.

So this is starting to sound a lot like the Mediterranean diet that we've already discussed, I do think that's a good place to start.

In addition though, fermented foods like kombucha, sauerkraut, miso, etc. and foods with cultures of bacteria already in them like yoghurt and kefir are helpful. And bitter foods like rocket and chicory are also good as among other things, they can trigger the digestion pathway, stimulating the saliva and gastric acid to be produced.

Pre and probiotics

So we talked a bit about soluble fibre being a prebiotic. Anything that helps the good gut bacteria thrive qualifies as a prebiotic; when you think about it, oestrogen itself is a prebiotic and all those complex carbohydrates are prebiotics. You can buy 'ready-made' prebiotics too, I often advise women to buy one which sorts out constipation and improves the biome, just to get things kick started.

Probiotics are live bacteria similar to some of those in your gut lining, an example is the added cultures in your yoghurt. The downside of your yoghurt is that some of those bacteria will be killed off in the stomach by the acid and so a smaller amount reaches the intestine. You can buy probiotics which can survive the acid and then turn up unscathed in the large intestine to do their job. There are LOADS on the market. You may well have taken them already e.g. after a course of antibiotics or when travelling abroad. It seems that you can use them to reset your biome. I haven't explored this yet as I'm trying to eat my biome better but I'll update you if I change my mind on that.

Fasting

Fasting boosts the microbiome, it appears that your Akkamansia particularly like a little time out. They do a bit of background spring cleaning so that they can return to the job fully refreshed and in full fitness. At least 12 hours without food is good and more is even better.

Exercise

This helps with the microbiome - I can't find anything definitive on the hows but there is an increase in the production of butyrate by the microbiome which in turn leads to less gut leakiness and all the other beneficial metabolic changes that we've already mentioned.

Exercise can also reduce the amount of stress chemicals flooding around the system which brings me to the next on the list.

<u>Reduce your response to stress</u> (I cover this more in the mood and heart chapters).

Stress has a direct impact on the lining of the gut leading to increased toxins leaking into the bloodstream. By changing the way we respond to stressors, we should be able to keep our microbiome protected.

Emotional and gut resilience all in one hit.

So, deep breaths at my end. I am loving all of this. I am a fan of anything that puts the opportunity for better health firmly back in our own hands and I, for one, am changing my diet (and stealthily that of my partner's) so that we can start looking ten years younger like all those people who live in Blue Zones. I want our house to be a Blue Zone.

What's a Blue Zone I hear you ask?! '...It's a region in the world where a higher than usual number of people live much longer than average...' I've just lifted that directly from Wikipedia. Think Okinawa in Japan where those beautiful women are still pearl fishing at 100 years of age.

I heard on a podcast but haven't found a back up study, that a 90-year-old living in a Blue Zone has the microbiome diversity of that of a 30-year-old...wow.

It seems Hippocrates, the father of medicine, was way ahead of his time with his 'You are what you eat' chat...

(I don't really like mentioning fathers of something without balancing things with a mother act. Henrietta Lacks is beautifully and rightly named as the 'mother of modern medicine'. Please read about her, I've popped some information at the end.)

So much on sleep!

Seriously, now those sleep scientists have started sharing their knowledge. It turns out that sleep is like some sort of cure-all for health, and lack of it is associated with a bunch of pretty significant changes to your system.

Lack of sleep can affect your immune system, make you more likely to become overweight, stressed, diabetic, have blood pressure problems, get Alzheimer's and a bunch of other stuff that we'll come to.

The studies are amazing for showing what sleep deprivation can cause...having six hours sleep the night before leaves your reaction times the same as if you'd just drunk three bottles of beer in the preceding half hour. Seriously! It wouldn't cross our minds to drive after three bottles of beer but plenty of people would happily do so after six hours sleep...I mean, sometimes you simply have to, work still has to happen, the kids still need to get to school and so on.

So here you are in your menopause and your sleep is all over the shop and you're now panicking because you're looking at my terrifying list above and that's making you feel even more anxious about your lack of sleep. Sorry.

Why is sleep affected in the menopause? Well, a lot is secondary to those pesky hot flushes and sweats, as although they can arrive at any time they fancy, they do prefer night time outings.

Oestrogen, throughout the usual period cycle, helps to lower the body temperature overnight (which is a good thing for sleep) and when we have less of it during our period (when oestrogen levels fall) we tend to be hotter...which fits with the fact that you often do want to throw the covers off when you're menstruating.

Progesterone, which you are now also missing, seems to have a boosting effect on one of the chemicals beneficial within the complex pathway of sleep. It is also thought to have an effect on the upper airway muscles and lack of progesterone may be part of the reason that post-menopausal women seem to develop sleep apnoea at an increased rate. This is when there are pauses in the breathing pattern which in turn can lead to fatigue and daytime sleepiness in addition to other problems. I thought this would be related to the weight gain of the menopause, but it appears to be independent of that (although weight gain does make it worse too).

Sleep is affected in three different ways - lots of waking through the night because of flushes and sweats, difficulty getting to sleep and waking early hours and not being able to get back to sleep.

My current sleep guru of choice is Professor Matthew Walker, who is a Brit working out of Berkeley University in California. He seems to have made sharing sleep information something of a mission. I've popped his book reference at the end if you would like to read it yourself. It makes sober but interesting reading.

So, in no particular order, good quality sleep helps:

- Keep your immune system healthy (people who were sleep deprived in the week before they had their flu vaccination had a significantly less effective response to it...worth thinking about if you're reading this in Covid times and your appointment for your vaccination is pending.)

- Reduce insulin resistance (more about this in the weight chapter) so helps in turn in keeping a normal body weight and glucose levels stable.

- Lower your heart rate and thence your blood pressure.

- Increase the 'I'm feeling full' chemical, whilst reducing the one that makes you think you need to eat more (and, because of lack of sleep, that extra eating isn't more kale but more pizza and ice cream). Poor sleepers can eat an extra 250-400 calories a day...I would have seriously skewed this study as I can eat an extra 250 calories in the space of a heartbeat and then a few more hundred again.

- Lay down memories and therefore open up space for more learning.

- Improve complex problem solving.

- Allow the brain to detox overnight (it's like a cleaning crew turns up and gives the brain a right old wash out, notably clearing one of the proteins, which if it accumulates, is associated with Alzheimer's).

- Allows the prefrontal cortex in the brain to regulate (damp down) our flight and fight responses and so reduce anxiety and emotional ups and downs.

- And more...

Given that the menopause is trying its very best to fight this good quality sleep, is it surprising that we get brain fog, reduced concentration and memory problems? Or that we're becoming more anxious and keyed up? Not so much.

Don't get me wrong, there are other reasons for these symptoms too so even menopausal women with good sleep and no flushes can still get the memory problems, mood swings and weight gain; but as I mentioned at the start, I think of this as part of the 'vicious circle symptoms' - as one thing goes out of kilter, it makes something else that's also going out of kilter worse.

What's recommended as a good night's sleep? Well, various souls list 7-9 hours although your man above says 8. The quality of the sleep is important, so you might get 8 hours but if you've been waking a lot through the night then it may not qualify as good.

Sadly, he says that you can't bank sleep, i.e. sleep more at the weekend to make up for rubbish sleep in the week. Also if you nap daily for fifteen minutes and that's normal for you then that's fine; but a nap here and there, to play catch up, doesn't really work beyond a slight improvement in your reaction time. It appears we build up a 'need' to sleep through the day and if we take an unexpected nap then we flush away some of that banked need.

What recommendations for improving your sleep? Well, let's lead out with the menopause specific ones and then the 'work for all' ones.

- Try to reduce those flushes (head back to the flushes chapter if you haven't visited there already.) Reduce your triggers...I know I keep repeating this but try a symptom tracker. A friend of mine recently found that on the nights that she had a single glass of wine, she couldn't get to sleep until 3 in the morning and yet she was fine with an occasional beer.

- Single duvets if you share a bed.

- If you wear clothing in bed, then leave a set close by to change into when the sweat hits.

- Consider sleeping on a towel so you can chuck this to the side, once the sweat has passed. I couldn't write this without thinking of the Princess and the Pea fairytale - menopausal women sleeping five foot above their mattress with about thirty towels beneath them ready to cast one aside with each sweat.

Then, in addition, good for all:

- Keep the room cool.

- Go to bed at the same time, wake at the same time...every day. Now hand on heart, I love a lie in, the weekend is not a weekend unless I can still be loafing around in my bed, drinking coffee (decaf...) and reading, etc. You can still do this but just wake up at the same time as you would in the week. I've had to train myself to do this and I do still slip and take an extra hour sometimes, but generally I try and keep to it, and it works. It's something called social jet lag, so if you sleep until 9am on Sunday instead of your usual 7am, you won't want to go to sleep at your usual time on Sunday evening because you're not ready to sleep.

- The bed is for sex and sleeping...I struggle with this one as I do tend to read a few pages before heading to sleep.

- However, it does lead to the next recommendation, that is, if you've been lying awake for more than 15 - 20 minutes then leave the bed and bedroom and head to another place to sit quietly in dim light, maybe read the dullest book known to man and then head back when you feel tired again. (I did write 'seed catalogue' instead of 'dull book' first, but realised that I am now at the age where the seed catalogue can totally flip me into a hyper-arousal state...)

- Practice acceptance - hmm, this one made me smile...it is really difficult to feel accepting about missing out on your sleep when you know you have a patient list of 30 people the following day. However, I do think I know how this translates into practice. I heard about sleeping for one and half hour blocks and as long as you got five of these blocks in, then you were all good. I'm not even sure where I heard this and I can't seem to find it anywhere now, but it really worked for me, as when I'd wake at four, I'd think 'hey, that's OK as I've already had 'x' blocks of sleep and I'm sure I'll get another one in before I have to be up...', and do you know what? I did.

- Meditation - some people say meditation in the day is best, as the worst thing for sleep is a hyper-arousal state and if you're beating yourself up for your mind wandering then that's not going to really add to your general sleepiness. With my yoga teacher hat on, I'd say learn to meditate in the day (congratulate yourself for noticing your mind wandering, but bring it back on track) and once you've got it sussed then a short meditation before bed or visualisation in the middle of the night is grand. Come find me at my yoga site if you'd like to learn more.

- Don't exercise too late (good sleep comes when the heart rate slows right down and exercising can interfere with that process).

- Avoid caffeine - a stimulant - after midday according to the Science of Sleep...I think my partner must be one of those people who metabolise caffeine differently from most - it has totally no effect on him and honestly, is his only form of hydration. Some people say that they're not affected by caffeine before bed, but in fact they are, it's affected their sleep quality but not their dropping off to sleep.

- Avoid/reduce alcohol - whilst alcohol is a sedative, it interferes with the way you sleep, so you might get to sleep quickly but the type of sleep you have will be less good.

- Keep the room dark or wear an eye mask.

- Get fit, stay fit, aim for a healthy weight and eat well - this advice turns up in pretty much every chapter I'm afraid, and I know it's not easy to do, but please stick with me.

And then if the above isn't working or not all of the time, seek out CBTi - Cognitive Behaviour Therapy for Insomnia.

This is a tried and tested method for treating insomnia, no matter whether this is menopause related or not, and in some countries and areas this can be available free from your health provider, so go online and check out some of the apps; most let you know if this is supported by your local health provider or not. It is a long-term solution for a problem that it really makes sense to solve.

Mood

Okey dokey, on to mood.

This time can be an emotional rollercoaster of tears, anger, irritability, anxiety and fear. You can be the life and soul of the party one minute and crying in the corner the next; calm one moment, screaming at everyone around you a moment later. Sound familiar?

Low mood and emotional triggering

So what about feeling blue? This is probably the least surprising of the headspace symptoms, as we already know that women suffer from premenstrual syndrome and postnatal depression, both of which are hormone related. How does this translate into symptoms at the menopause?

In the SWAN study about 50% of women complained of at least one 'negative mood' symptom for 1-5 days out of the preceding two weeks: feeling blue or depressed, irritability or grouchiness (I love the word grouchy), feeling tense or nervous, or frequent mood changes.

Good to know it's not just you, but here's the thing…you've spent years carefully cultivating your cool, approachable, 'take it as it comes' female boss persona, only to have it come crashing to the ground when you burst into tears every time your colleague shares a kitten video or you can't make the charger plug fit in your laptop.

Now, I've always been someone who cries at Lassie movies. I think easy tears in emotionally uncharged situations is my brain's housekeeping solution for coping with all the life that passes through my surgery. Whilst there have been rare times that I've cried with patients, generally it is better that I'm on the scooping up end of that emotion and able to think clearly about what best to offer next. So Lassie, anything by David Attenborough and the brilliant Repair shop all lead to Olympic level blubbering at my end, just letting all that suppressed emotion out. But this got worse…

How do you know when your low mood is menopause and not actual depression?

When you do the The Greene Climacteric Symptom Score, you'll see that it does categorise symptoms into groups and one of those are the 'depression' symptoms. If you score over 10 in that domain, then it is more likely you're depressed than suffering the mood changes related to changing hormones. I've popped a link to this on the resource sheet.

If your low mood is impacting on your daily activities e.g. getting up, getting dressed, meeting people, going to work, then it is more likely that you're suffering from depression and would benefit from seeking help.

So, definitely a good one to check in with your counsellor or doctor about. You may be surprised, depression has many very physical symptoms e.g. fatigue, that we don't think of as mental health markers.

Anxiousness

Anxiety is something that came as a bolt out of the blue for me. I hadn't had any change in my bleed cycle when it arrived so it was even more difficult to categorise as perimenopause related.

I've not really been an anxious person before this, I've had all the usual female concerns - low self-esteem, happy days and sad days but anxiety, not a sliver. I've always pretty much followed the Dalai Lama's creed, if it's a problem you can do something about, then do it and don't worry about it, and if you can't do something about it, then there's nothing to be gained from worrying about it.

But all of a sudden I'm sweating the small stuff, and not doing the usual things I'd want to do - single track downhill mountain biking, I was never good at it, but it became a horror field of likely injury so I stopped doing it altogether. Anxiety about my partner's health, my family's health, my health and so the list went on.

What do we mean by anxiety? Well, it's the worry symptoms, that feeling of ill ease, that things are spinning out of our control. We all get it at times e.g. before an exam, but when it gets out of hand it can get in the way of living a normal life.

And the thing is not all doctors know that this can be a perimenopause symptom either. I was at a GP conference where they update you on guidelines and changes in research. I really admire the person who was running this particular course, but when they came to the menopause update, they downplayed the anxiety symptom saying that they didn't think that was truly menopause at all. Of course, I was so anxious that they might be right that I didn't challenge them on it!

Again, how do you know when your anxiousness has tipped over into an anxiety disorder?

The Greene Climacteric Symptom Scale does differentiate between what might be more than usual anxiousness of the menopause and anxiety itself, so take a quick look at the resource sheet and fill in the form and go from there.

If anxiety is starting to interfere with daily life, then seek out advice from your doctor or counsellor.

What to do?

Both problems, whilst different, can generally benefit from the same advice.

- Try to get that sleep in - lack of sleep has its own deleterious effect on mood.

- Reduce alcohol - this can often be reached for as a self-medication, a nice glass of wine at the end of a stressful day; however alcohol can mimic and increase the symptoms of depression. It is a happy-making drug for moments and a sad-making drug ongoing.

- Eat well - the microbiome is also thought to influence mood (see the Gut chapter). This is still early days for this research but it's exciting to imagine that we can eat ourselves happier and less anxious.

- Exercise regularly - according to a Cochrane review (Cochrane reviews look at multiple research studies and pool the information together to get a result) exercise is better than no treatment at all for improving mood.

- Share how you're feeling - your partner thinks they've done something wrong (they may have but let's put that aside for a moment); you're not quite so touchy-feely, you're irritable when previously you've been tolerant. They don't really know what to make of it. It's worth talking about, not all day and all night but a 'hey, this is what's happening and this is how I feel.' Maybe try to get your partner to read at least the chapter on mood and anxiety and the one on sex, sometimes it's an easier place to start a conversation from...like a menopause book club for couples.

Cognitive Behaviour Therapy (CBT) is a proven way of treating low mood and anxiety and is often available through your local counselling services. In fact there is now online CBT which means you can do this from the comfort of your own home. You may be able to access this without making an appointment with your doctor. I've put a couple of book recommendations at the end that you may find helpful.

Mindfulness and Meditation are starting to find traction for treating mood. Another Cochrane review showed that relaxation techniques are effective, so that's a good place to start. There's loads of resources around at the moment (particularly in view of the low mood and anxiety increase with the pandemic) and I'll list a few favourites at the end.

Yoga, yoga and yoga...ooh by the way, did I mention yoga?

Heart disease

I don't know about you, but when I think of female diseases I tend to think about the cancers. I have three friends who have had breast cancer but only one who has had a heart attack and she's 70.

When it comes to what women might die of though, heart disease is tops. The Centre for Disease Control and Prevention (CDC) figures in 2017 showed that heart disease was the number one cause of death for women in the US, causing about 1 in every 5 female deaths.

We tend to think of this as one for the boys, but that's just because we've been partially protected until the menopause. The rate of heart disease in women suddenly takes off after the menopause until the point where we actually overtake men in terms of numbers of souls with it.

Women who have diabetes, raised blood pressure (hypertension), raised central abdominal weight, abnormal cholesterol and triglyceride (lipids) profiles and smokers are particularly at risk of heart disease. Any of those look familiar? According to one review

159

paper I read '...80% of midlife women have one or more cardiac risk factors...'. I expect you already know how I'm going to tail-end this chapter...sorry!

Let's get into the background.

When we talk about Ischaemic heart disease (IHD), what we mean is that not enough oxygenated blood is getting to the heart muscle.

There are two main reasons for reduced blood flow to the heart - the vessels supplying it can be narrowed or they can go into spasm (which means they tighten up).

Traditionally when we've talked about coronary artery or coronary heart disease, we've been referring to atherosclerosis. This is when a fatty deposit builds up on the lining of the arteries and leads to narrowing of the arteries. This reduces the amount of oxygenated blood that can get to the muscle of the heart, but also it can lead to small clots of blood forming on the deposit; these can break off and travel down the artery until the vessel is blocked off completely. The tissue beyond, in this case the heart muscle, dies from lack of oxygen

160

- this is a heart attack. (This can happen with the brain too and that's the cause of the more common type of stroke).

Atherosclerosis can be confirmed on a coronary angiogram which, via tracking a radioactive dye, shows where the narrowings are in the main arteries of the heart.

More and more work is being done on women with heart disease which shows that this traditional picture of heart disease isn't the whole shebang. Yes, women can get atherosclerosis, but women can also have ischaemic heart disease and a normal coronary angiogram.

Which brings us to the spasm. It appears that women may suffer more 'microvascular' heart disease - these are the very small blood vessels of the heart, which don't show on our traditional angiograms.

There seems to be more reactivity within these vessels (spasm or tightening of the arteries.) This is thought to be the mechanism behind migraines (migraine is now one of the risk factors which we use when we do a Qrisk calculation to work out who might get heart disease) and is certainly what's happening in Raynaud's (when the fingers and toes go white with exposure to cold); both of which appear more often in women.

We've talked about the elasticity of many tissues being affected by loss of oestrogen - the skin, the vagina and so it's not surprising to consider that the blood vessels are also affected because they're made of elastin and collagen too. The result is that they become stiffer.

In addition to all of the above:

An inflammatory marker called C-Reactive Protein (CRP) is on average higher in women than in men (this isn't a menopause change, this is seen from the start of periods onwards). A number of inflammatory diseases like rheumatoid arthritis and lupus are seen much more frequently in women. Rising CRP seems to match with rising risk of heart disease...

The cholesterol and triglycerides (lipids) change after the menopause. The 'good' HDL cholesterol reduces, the total cholesterol rises and a subset of 'bad' LDL cholesterol rises. The triglycerides (which traditionally no one has really paid too much attention to unless they're obscenely high) can rise and these seem to have much more of an impact on women than they do for men. All together this is called dyslipidaemia and it is more likely to cause atherosclerosis.

What does this mean in practice?

Given the above differences in cause, it will come as no surprise that women often don't present with the cardinal symptom of coronary heart disease - central chest pain with exercise.

Women may get more jaw pain, symptoms at rest, shortness of breath and new onset tiredness and so may be overlooked as having heart problems at all. Their investigations may be directed elsewhere and if they do end up with cardiac investigations, the results may be normal even when heart disease is present. Tough times.

The Qrisk calculator, which I referred to earlier, is a starting point for recognising if you are at risk but be aware, if you're reading this outside the UK, that it looks at a UK population only so may not be relevant to you. There are also calculators that show you how much difference your own changes can make to this e.g. if you give up smoking.

I feel a bit of a ratbag going down the route of lifestyle changes again, you're probably getting a bit frustrated with hearing about them by now. I'm hoping lots of you are reading this in the perimenopause period (or even before) so that you have the chance to prevent rather than having to chase.

I'm talking in terms of primary prevention - things you can do to reduce your risk of getting heart disease. (Secondary prevention is when you've already got a problem and you aim to reduce its impact, e.g. someone who's had a heart attack being advised to take aspirin).

Nutrition choices and weight loss

Try to reduce the central weight gain - and don't forget the 'skinny' person with visceral fat. I've talked about vicious circle symptoms, I feel that now I'm writing a vicious circle book where I keep directing you back to the weight chapter. Again, it's not how much you eat (although that does count), the focus is more on what you eat.

Exercise

There is lots of excellent evidence to show that exercise and weight/resistance training reduce your risk of getting heart disease.

According to the Cochrane study 'Exercise for people with high cardiovascular risk', exercise can reduce blood pressure, increase good cholesterol whilst reducing the bad, and reduce the triglycerides. It helps with weight loss, improves the blood insulin and glucose and makes us feel happy. It is thought to improve the blood vessel function and reduce those inflammatory markers.

We've all heard for many years about the benefits of cardio exercise - the running, swimming, walking, etc. but now there is good evidence to show that weight or resistance training is also good at reducing heart disease by scooping up the sugar and the triglycerides into the muscles.

Reduce Stress

And no surprises, stress increases heart disease. So we need to reduce this...hmm.

You've undoubtedly heard talk about our 'flight and fight' system; this is no longer being used to save our lives by kicking in when we have to outrun that much maligned sabre tooth tiger, instead it's working when we stress out over a deadline or are stuck in a traffic jam, late for a meeting. This leads to a body bathed in cortisol, adrenaline and noradrenaline, all having their own impact on heart health.

It makes sense to reduce stressors, but honestly, sometimes we simply can't - we have to work, we may not have many choices in the

166

job market, we can't suddenly give away three kids because we've realised that two was probably as many as we could financially afford. Sometimes life is stressful and our lack of ability to make a change to it is also stressful.

Instead we have to retrain ourselves to deal with stress in a different way - make it less impactful, essentially give it less of a starring role in our lives. This is where Cognitive Behaviour Therapy, mindfulness, meditation, Tai Chi, yoga and exercise all come in.

Yoga...there it is again...I should have set a 'yoga bingo' challenge at the start, first to full house gets a prize. This time I've managed to find a Cochrane review to partially back the yoga claim up!!

'...The results showed that yoga has favourable effects on diastolic blood pressure, high-density lipoprotein (HDL) cholesterol and triglycerides (a blood lipid), and uncertain effects on low-density lipoprotein (LDL) cholesterol...'

Ha! Anyway, these were small, short duration trials that fed into this review but better quality research often comes off the back of these smaller studies. Let's hope so, keep me in a job after I've retired from the medical coalface.

Heart disease - this is a massive subject. It needs to be, it is the number one killer of men and women, and there is so much more research and understanding to come; hopefully with specific focus on women rather than lumping us together with men in one big, amorphous heart disease pot.

Until then if we can start improving the elements over which we have some control, then hopefully we'll live long enough to add new things to our armoury as more research filters through.

Fatigue

It's a shame you can't pop a GIF into an eBook as I have a favourite which just about sums up menopausal fatigue. It's of a three-ish-year-old girl who's leaning against the side of a bed, and the look of utter frustration that she can't stay awake a moment longer is written all over her face; she has that 'just tipping into tears' look about her. I'll see if I can pop it up on Facebook.

Menopausal fatigue is like no other. It is exactly what it says on the tin, a complete lack of energy to do more than lie flat.

You push yourself to get up and do stuff and that helps but inside you're that little girl, frustrated and annoyed that overnight you seem to have suddenly just 'got old'.

After reading to this point, it would be somewhat surprising not to have fatigue on the list of symptoms, we've dealt with plenty of things that could be causing it:

169

Disturbed sleep

Joint pain (being in pain is knackering)

Urinary frequency - particularly having to get up at night

Increased weight - meaning each step feels like you're carrying shopping bags full of kilos.

Reduced muscle mass making each task more difficult

Joylessness - the low mood/lack of happiness can often translate into a feeling of fatigue.

Anxiousness -those fight and flight chemicals racing around can make the body feel like it's run a marathon.

And on the list goes.

The understanding of the menopause is still, slightly surprisingly, in its early days. The interplay of the sex hormones in so many other pathways will likely lead to other discoveries to explain why fatigue is such a major part of the menopause in addition to the reasons above.

I shall keep reading to stay abreast of this, as it will likely then filter into additional treatment offerings and advice.

Until then, I guess the usual recommendations apply...check in with your doctor to make sure that it's menopause fatigue, then recognise which of the symptoms is the likely majority shareholder in your fatigue and take that on first.

If it's loss of sleep then aim to set that right and then see what's left over and tackle that.

It is beyond annoying, I went from someone who could do a bunch of stuff in one day to doing significantly less; it really does feel as if someone turned on a tap and drained you dry of all your energy.

It is quite difficult to work out if you're depressed or unmotivated or menopausal or what on earth is going on, but as I say, take small steps to improve aspects and hopefully things will turn a corner. You're not alone - one study showed that 85.3% of post-menopausal women and 46.5% of peri-menopausal women reported symptoms of physical and mental exhaustion compared to just 19.7% of the pre-menopausal women.

What's the benefit of knowing that? Well, it's all part of what they call practising acceptance (grrrrrrr....). I loathe being tired much of the time, but I'm not making it any easier on myself by getting angry and frustrated and expending all those extra energy points on senseless unhappiness. I can 'accept' that I'm part of a team of 85.3% post-menopausal women who feel like this and then crack on and try and do my bit to turn it around. I can be gracious to myself as fatigue is a 'menopause thing' not a 'me thing'.

Easier said than done...believe me!

What treatments are there?

So you've read to this point, maybe you've already instituted some of the lifestyle changes and have better control over your flushes, and now you're thinking about what else there might be to add.

You'd like to know if there are medications or complementary treatments that will offset some of the problems we've been discussing and maybe even protect you against osteoporosis and heart disease.

I wrote this book to alert you to the changes that the menopause brings and help you feel in control by having a greater understanding thereof. The treatments that you can use are another book's worth of information. (If enough of you e-mail me to say you'd like to hear more (in this style) then I'm happy to crack on and do that.)

Here is what I will say though.

No one size fits all. Women are joyfully, amazingly different in ways beyond the surface characteristics. What floats my boat as a tool of change may leave you entirely cold, and I may raise a quizzical eyebrow at some of the choices that you may be considering pursuing. However, if you don't choose something that resonates with you then likelihood is that it won't feel comfortable and it won't make a difference.

For instance, I love the concept of Ayurveda - particularly as it allows for Western medicine to run alongside. (In fact, I think I've just set myself the task of training therein...you were here for the light switch moment!) I find working alongside complementary therapists rewarding, learning an enormous amount from them and I think the opportunity to share the space of wellbeing is exciting. There are fantastic menopause specialists out there and your wonderful family doctor is happy to get involved and support you.

As long as who you choose isn't into snake oil sales then anyone who can support you in this journey is good. You've chosen them and that means that something about what they offer makes sense to you, and therefore you're already part-way on the path to success.

How do you know if someone is selling snake oil? You may not, but I think that if you are seeking a change e.g. a reduction in hot flushes, then it's worth setting a date for when you'd expect to see the improvement and if it hasn't happened then maybe think about a different treatment or provider.

For instance, if you came to see me in my clinic asking to start HRT (and there were no reasons not to) I'd advise that you'd see a good benefit from it at about three months. If you were seeing me as a menopause coach and had followed all the lifestyle plans we'd agreed together and hadn't seen positive change by three months, I would be recommending that you look for another pathway of support.

I'm sure some interventions take longer to see an effect, but what I'm recommending is that you get a sense from the provider about 'how long before I see change', and then set a review date accordingly.

So, what else *is* out there?

Hormone Replacement Therapy (HRT)

This is the opportunity to replace the missing hormones, either by tablet, patch, gel and - a new one to the market - spray.

I have two things I will say about HRT at this juncture:

The first is a prescribing issue - if you have a uterus, you *must* have progesterone in addition to the oestrogen. Using oestrogen alone long term can lead to thickening of the lining of the womb and can, in some cases, eventually lead to cancer. The progesterone can be in a coil, patch, tablet or vaginal capsule.

The second is a risk issue - if you are going to start HRT, it is recommended that you start within ten years of your menopause. After this point you may well have established heart disease and this may lead to an increased risk of heart problems rather than reducing the risk.

If you're unsure about HRT then 'Oestrogen Matters' is a comprehensive book about the research. It is a love letter to HRT which is good as it resets the pendulum swing that has made HRT the villain in recent years.

The Menopause societies who I list on the resource sheet are also excellent repositories of the most up to date information in terms of risk/benefit ratio. There are also some terrific doctor-led websites and resources too.

Non - HRT medications

Doctors can prescribe other drugs to help with some of the symptoms of the menopause e.g. SSRIs, this is a medication group usually used for depression and anxiety but can be used to help with flushes. I have put links to the main menopause societies who list the information on these.

<u>Herbal and nutritional supplements</u>

Again there are some very good leaflets on the menopause society websites with recommendations about what may be helpful and what you should take care with.

We touched on the benefits of some nutritional changes within the microbiome chapter and sometimes pre and probiotics may help fast track improvement whilst making the dietary changes to ensure gut health recovers.

Wine, gin and me

I just couldn't go without talking about wine. I love it, always have (well, always is probably pushing it, I expect there was a short time in infancy when it wasn't my bag).

I also love a good G and T in the summer and a beer when I come off the water, but for me wine is where it's at. We're not talking much wine I hasten to add, just in case you disregard the previous however many pages because I am now in your eyes 'a drinker', but a glass or two here and there.

So it was all a bit upsetting when I found I could no longer drink it. It either caused me to flush or it had me up pretty much all the night. Other menopausal friends report similar - headaches, bad night's sleep and excessive fatigue. To be honest, gin isn't great either...beer seems to be my only friend.

I have a pal, who went through her perimenopause some years before me and she would tell us that she '...*can only drink champagne...*'. Now at that time I was premenopausal and simply thought that this was a brilliant ruse for just drinking champagne; but do you know what, she was right!

Because I'm a scientist at heart, I refused to believe that *all* wine was the problem and so I have selflessly tried out a few different ones for you. It seems organic is good, bottled at source is good and yes, champagne is good!

And don't you just love women? There are a bunch of female entrepreneurs out there who have also hit the 'wine is poison' part of the menopause and have simply created new businesses making wines and spirits to suit the perimenopausal lady...I have yet to try some but, once again, in the interests of 'science' and in order to serve you all well, I will aim to take on this thankless task.

Whine over!

Signing off

I think this is where I sign off; thank you for joining me on this journey! I think that this is such an important topic for me because I like to see women thrive and to be honest, I like to thrive myself.

I remember, way back in the day when I was a med student, a friend's Mum hiving me off into a corner to ask if 'she was losing her mind'. She was waking in the middle of the night, overwhelmed with feelings of anxiety and having to go out into the garden, hyperventilating and bathed in sweat; she didn't know what was going on and felt unable to talk to her friends or her doctor. It felt nice being able to reassure her that this was her hormones and as difficult as this stage was, it would pass (albeit, that at the time, I didn't know quite how long that might take! When you're a medical student you're happy with the small wins.)

I have experienced most of that hideous list of symptoms at some stage along the way and my wonderful husband deserves an award for riding the menopause waves with me. A friend of mine overheard him at a party a few years ago giving his mates a 'heads up on what's happening next' chat...cue lots of downcast faces.

I have watched marriages dissolve, perfectly good jobs thrown in and plenty of anguish related to the transition that is the menopause; it would make me happy if I knew that your understanding of the symptoms in some way offset any of the above. As I said at the start, I truly believe that the more you understand and own a problem, the easier it is to live with.

I would love to hear your thoughts on this book and if you'd like to hear from me on specific topics.

I will be updating my Instagram erratically (I came late to social media and I think we can safely say, it's not my most comfortable space) and if I do learn something HUGE, I'll probably update there and if I get savvy via a blog. You can tell I'm hedging my updating bets at the moment ;-).

Take great, great care and continue to live your best, occasionally sweaty, 'fretty' life.

Louise   xxx

Please feel free to feedback, I'll try and find some way of sharing a link via the paperback. If you feel able to offer a bite sized review, then I'd love to hear it. You don't have to leave any identifiers but for those of you who would like it, I have put a short guided meditation that can be downloaded directly, to say thank you. I'll email irregularly if I have a workshop or something useful menopause-wise pending, so please indicate on the form if you'd like to join my mailing list. I'm @yourmidlifemagic on instagram and the same on Facebook.

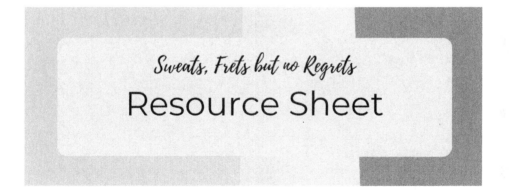

Sweats, Frets but no Regrets

Resource Sheet

So I haven't quite worked out how best to share the resource sheet for paperback. I've opened out the links now that you can't just click on them. I'll work on this though and hopefully update via my sales page.

You can follow me on instagram (@yourmidlifemagic) or Facebook at Your Midlife Magic (I have absolutely no idea how to put a link in for that...I'll work up to it!) and I'll update as I find new things out.

My website is www.yourmidlifemagic.com

My yoga website is www.yogafor.co.uk

Contraception

If you go through your menopause pre-50, the advice is to use contraception for two years after the last period. If you go through your menopause post 50 then the recommendation is for one year after your last period. Current 2021.

Symptoms

Balance menopause support app

Greene Climacteric scale questionnaire

https://www.menopausematters.co.uk/greenescore.php

N.B.

Clinically Anxious = Anxiety Score of 10 or more

Clinically Depressed = Depression Score of 10 or more

The physiology of the menstrual cycle

https://teachmephysiology.com/reproductive-system/development-maturation/menstrual-cycle/

Sleep

Science of Sleep - Prof Matthew Walker

Osteoporosis

FRAX score

https://www.sheffield.ac.uk/FRAX/tool.aspx?country=1

Calcium calculator

https://www.cgem.ed.ac.uk/research/rheumatological/calcium-calculator/

Nutrition

Weight

- BMI calculator
- https://www.nhs.uk/live-well/healthy-weight/bmi-calculator/

- Waist height ratio
- https://www.coventrywarksapc.nhs.uk/Calculators/Waist-to-Height-Ratio

- Waist measurement NHS
- https://www.nhs.uk/common-health-questions/lifestyle/why-is-my-waist-size-important/

The Eight week blood sugar diet - Dr Michael Mosley

European Journal of Nutrition 100 richest dietary sources of phenol
https://www.nature.com/articles/ejcn2010221

The Diet Myth - Professor Tim Spector

The Clever Guts Diet recipe book - Dr Clare Bailey

The Fast 800 - Dr Michael Mosley

Hot flushes

Managing hot flushes and Night sweats - CBT self help guide to the menopause - Myra Hunter and Melanie Smith

Pelvic floor

https://www.squeezyapp.com/

https://www.nafc.org/kegel-exercises

www.bladdermatters.co.uk

Genitourinary syndrome of the Menopause

Lubricants

https://www.tandfonline.com/doi/full/10.3109/13697137.2015.1124259?sr c=

The table of pH and osmolality of lubricants and moisturisers is in the middle of this paper. Scroll down if you don't want to read the rest of it.

Eyes

https://www.bsuh.nhs.uk/wp-content/uploads/sites/5/2016/09/dry-eye s.pdf

Mood

Overcoming Anxiety: A Self-help Guide to Using CBT - Helen Kennerley

Breathing Exercises

https://www.guysandstthomas.nhs.uk/resources/patient-information/therapies/abdominal-breathing.pdf

Feeling Great - David Burns

Feeling Good - David Burns (his previous iteration but might be a bit cheaper)

http://getselfhelp.co.uk/ is a very tired looking website (perimenopausal maybe?) but was recommended to me by a colleague who is now a CBT therapist. It seems like an excellent resource with lots of free downloadable information and self help guidance.

Skin

The Positive Ageing Plan - Dr Vicky Dondos

Treatments

Non HRT medications for symptoms
https://www.menopausematters.co.uk/prescribed.php

Complementary therapies for treatment

https://www.womens-health-concern.org/help-and-advice/factsheets/complementaryalternative-therapies-menopausal-women/

HRT

https://www.womens-health-concern.org/help-and-advice/factsheets/hrt-know-benefits-risks/

Also on HRT

Oestrogen Matters - Avrum Bluming and Carol Tavris

Menopause Societies

If you type menopause society into your search engine then you'll find those local to you. I've listed a few above. Some have their patient information leaflets on the same site or link you across to a different site.

These societies are 'on it', they update their guidance alongside new published research particularly on hormone replacement therapy.

British Menopause society

www.thebms.org.uk

189

www.menopausematters.co.uk

North American Menopause society

https://www.menopause.org/

Canadian Menopause society

https://www.sigmamenopause.com/

Doctors

There are some amazing doctors out there doing sterling work on keeping doctors and patients up to date.

I've only listed one below because she's in the UK and is therefore well known to me, but please update me with anyone in your area/country so I can keep adding to this resource list.

My menopause doctor

The information contained in this resource sheet is provided for general purposes only. It is not intended as and should not be relied upon as medical advice. The author is not responsible for any specific health needs that may require medical supervision. If you have underlying health problems or have any doubts about the advice contained in this book, you should contact a qualified medical or other appropriate professional.

References

Menopause: diagnosis, symptoms and management

https://www.sciencealert.com/beluga-whales-and-narwhals-go-through-menopause-new-study-finds

Harlow SD, Gass M, Hall JE, et al. Executive summary of the Stages of Reproductive Aging Workshop +10: addressing the unfinished agenda of staging reproductive aging. Climacteric. 2012;15(2):105-114.

Perlman, Barry; Kulak, David; Goldsmith, Laura T.; Weiss, Gerson The etiology of menopause: not just ovarian dysfunction but also a role for the central nervous system, Global Reproductive Health: June 2018 - Volume 3 - Issue 2 - p e8 doi: 10.1097/GRH.0000000000000008

NICE guideline [NG23]Published date: 12 November 2015 Last updated: 05 December 2019

2016 Ipsos MORI poll on behalf of the British Menopause Society
https://thebms.org.uk/wp-content/uploads/2020/09/BMS-NationalSur
vey-SEPT2020-B.pdf

Lösel R, Wehling M. Nongenomic actions of steroid hormones. Nat
Rev Mol Cell Biol. 2003 Jan;4(1):46-56. doi: 10.1038/nrm1009. PMID:
12511868.

Weight

Molly C. Carr, The Emergence of the Metabolic Syndrome with
Menopause, The Journal of Clinical Endocrinology & Metabolism,
Volume 88, Issue 6, 1 June 2003, Pages 2404–2411

Wilcox G. Insulin and insulin resistance. Clin Biochem Rev.
2005;26(2):19-39.

MonashUni - resources for healthcare practitioners: Insulin resistance

C V SB, S B, A S. Analysis of the degree of insulin resistance in post menopausal women by using skin temperature measurements and fasting insulin and fasting glucose levels: a case control study. J Clin Diagn Res. 2012;6(10):1644-1647.

Anisha A. Gupte, Henry J. Pownall, Dale J. Hamilton, "Estrogen: An Emerging Regulator of Insulin Action and Mitochondrial Function", Journal of Diabetes Research, vol. 2015, Article ID 916585, 9 pages, 2015.

Berg, G., Mesch, V. & Siseles, N. Abdominal Obesity and Metabolic Alterations in the Menopausal Transition. Curr Obstet Gynecol Rep 1, 63–70 (2012).

Wan-Yu Huang,Chia-Chu Chang,Dar-Ren Chen,Chew-Teng Kor,Ting-Yu Chen,Hung-Ming Wu Circulating leptin and adiponectin are associated with insulin resistance in healthy postmenopausal women with hot flashes Published: April 27, 2017

Gallo-Villegas, Jaime et al. Efficacy of high-intensity, low-volume interval training compared to continuous aerobic training on insulin resistance, skeletal muscle structure and function in adults with metabolic syndrome: study protocol for a randomized controlled clinical trial (Intraining-MET)." Trials vol. 19,1 144. 27 Feb. 2018

Cancer Research UK - Cancer risk statistics https://www.cancerresearchuk.org/health-professional/cancer-statistics/risk/overweight-and-obesity Jan 2021

Heart disease

WHO causes of death: https://www.who.int/news-room/fact-sheets/detail/the-top-10-causes-of-death

Women and Ischaemic Heart Disease Leslee J. Shaw, Raffaelle Bugiardini, C.Noel Bairey Merz Journal of the American College of Cardiology Vol 54, No. 17, 2009

Feldstein, C., Akopian, M., Renauld, A. et al. Insulin resistance and hypertension in postmenopausal women. J Hum Hypertens 16, S145–S150 (2002)

Dariush Mozaffarian, Peter W.F. Wilson, and William B. Kannel Beyond Established and Novel Risk Factors Lifestyle Risk Factors for Cardiovascular Disease CIRCULATIONAHA.107.738732Circulation. 2008;117:3031–3038

Hartley L, Dyakova M, Holmes J, Clarke A, Lee MS, Ernst E, Rees K. Yoga for the primary prevention of cardiovascular disease. Cochrane Database of Systematic Reviews 2014, Issue 5. Art. No.: CD010072. DOI: 10.1002/14651858.CD010072.pub2. Accessed 19 April 2021.

National Center for Health Statistics :Mortality Data on CDC WONDER

Underlying Cause-of-Death https://wonder.cdc.gov/mortsql.html

Genitourinary syndrome of the Menopause

196

Pelvic floor

Dumoulin C, Cacciari L, Hay-Smith EC. Pelvic floor muscle training versus no treatment, or inactive control treatments, for urinary incontinence in women. Cochrane Database of Systematic Reviews 2018, Issue 10. Art. No.: CD005654. DOI: 10.1002/14651858.CD005654.pub4

Vaginal lubricants

D. Edwards & N. Panay (2016) Treating vulvovaginal atrophy/genitourinary syndrome of menopause: how important is vaginal lubricant and moisturizer composition?, Climacteric, 19:2, 151-161, DOI: 10.3109/13697137.2015.1124259

Sexual health

Simson R v, Kulasegaram R. Sexual health and the older adult BMJ 2012; 344 :e688 doi:10.1136/sbmj.e688

Tanton C, Geary RS, Clifton S, et al Sexual health clinic attendance and non-attendance in Britain: findings from the third National Survey of Sexual Attitudes and Lifestyles (Natsal-3)Sexually Transmitted Infections 2018;94:268-276.

Public Health England. Sexually Transmitted Infections (STIs): Annual Data Tables. Table 8: Attendances by gender, sexual risk and age group, 2012 to 2016. 2017. https://www.gov.uk/government/statistics/sexually-transmitted-infections-stis-annual-data-tables.

Contraception

FSRH Clinical Guideline: Contraception for Women Aged over 40 Years Published on: 26 September 2019 Author: FSRH Clinical Effectiveness Unit

Brain stuff

Harvard Centre on the Developing Child - Executive function- lay interpretation.

2017 Edelman poll British Menopause Society National survey

Edwards, Hannaford MSc1; Duchesne, Annie PhD2; Au, April S. PhD1; Einstein, Gillian PhD1 The many menopauses: searching the cognitive research literature for menopause types, Menopause: January 2019 - Volume 26 - Issue 1 - p 45-65

McEwen BS, Akama KT, Spencer-Segal JL, Milner TA, Waters EM. Estrogen effects on the brain: actions beyond the hypothalamus via novel mechanisms. Behav Neurosci. 2012;126(1):4-16.

Gava, G.; Orsili, I.; Alvisi, S.; Mancini, I.; Seracchioli, R.; Meriggiola, M.C. Cognition, Mood and Sleep in Menopausal Transition: The Role of Menopause Hormone Therapy. Medicina 2019, 55, 668. https://doi.org/10.3390/medicina55100668

Karlamangla AS, Lachman ME, Han W, Huang M, Greendale GA (2017) Evidence for Cognitive Aging in Midlife Women: Study of Women's Health Across the Nation. PLOS ONE 12(1): e0169008

Mood and menopause: findings from the Study of Women's Health Across the Nation (SWAN) over 10 years Joyce T Bromberger 1, Howard M Kravitz Obstet Gynecol Clin North Am. 2011 Sep;38(3):609-25.

Frey BN, Lord C, Soares CN. Depression during menopausal transition: a review of treatment strategies and pathophysiological correlates. Menopause Int. 2008 Sep;14(3):123-8. doi: 10.1258/mi.2008.008019. PMID: 18714078.

SWAN Newsletter November 2000 Negative Mood and Depression https://www.swanstudy.org/wps/wp-content/uploads/2020/03/112000.pdf

Sleep

200

Gava, G.; Orsili, I.; Alvisi, S.; Mancini, I.; Seracchioli, R.; Meriggiola, M.C. Cognition, Mood and Sleep in Menopausal Transition: The Role of Menopause Hormone Therapy. Medicina 2019, 55, 668.

Matthew Walker Why we sleep- the new science of sleep and dreams

Jan Wesström Jan Ulfberg Staffan Nilsson Sleep apnea and hormone replacement therapy: a pilot study and a literature review, Acta Obstet Gynecol Scand 2005; 84: 54–57.

Eyal Shahar, Susan Redline, Terry Young, Lori L. Boland, Carol M. Baldwin, F. Javier Nieto, George T. O'Connor, David M. Rapoport, and John A. Robbins for the Sleep Heart Health Study Research Group Hormone Replacement Therapy and Sleep-disordered Breathing American Journal of Respiratory and Critical Care Medicine 2003; 167 1186-1192

MSK

Bay-Jensen AC, Tabassi NC, Sondergaard LV, et al. The response to oestrogen deprivation of the cartilage collagen degradation marker, CTX-II, is unique compared with other markers of collagen turnover. Arthritis Res Ther. 2009;11(1):R9. doi:10.1186/ar2596

Godfrey RJ, Madgwick Z, Whyte GP. The exercise-induced growth hormone response in athletes. Sports Med. 2003;33(8):599-613. doi: 10.2165/00007256-200333080-00005. PMID: 12797841.

Lowe, Dawn A.1; Baltgalvis, Kristen A.2; Greising, Sarah M.1 Mechanisms Behind Estrogen's Beneficial Effect on Muscle Strength in Females, Exercise and Sport Sciences Reviews: April 2010 - Volume 38 - Issue 2 - p 61-67 doi: 10.1097/JES.0b013e3181d496bc

Taylor J. Marcell, Review Article: Sarcopenia: Causes, Consequences, and Preventions, The Journals of Gerontology: Series A, Volume 58, Issue 10, October 2003, Pages M911–M916,

Howe TE, Shea B, Dawson LJ, Downie F, Murray A, Ross C, Harbour RT, Caldwell LM, Creed G. Exercise for preventing and treating
202

osteoporosis in postmenopausal women. Cochrane Database Syst Rev. 2011 Jul 6;(7):CD000333.

Osteoporosis Clinical Guidelines for prevention and treatment - Executive Summary; National Osteoporosis Guideline Group (NOGG) 2014 Fracture risk women vs men

Osteoporosis - Prevention of fragility fractures; NICE CKS, June 2015 (UK access only)

Föger-Samwald U, Dovjak P, Azizi-Semrad U, Kerschan-Schindl K, Pietschmann P. Osteoporosis: Pathophysiology and therapeutic options. EXCLI J. 2020;19:1017-1037. Published 2020 Jul 20. doi:10.17179/excli2020-2591

Bonaiuti D, Shea B, Iovine R, Negrini S, Robinson V, Kemper HC, Wells G, Tugwell P, Cranney A. Exercise for preventing and treating osteoporosis in postmenopausal women. Cochrane Database Syst Rev. 2002;(3):CD000333. Update in: Cochrane Database Syst Rev. 2011;(7):CD000333. PMID: 12137611.
203

Benedetti MG, Furlini G, Zati A, Letizia Mauro G. The Effectiveness of Physical Exercise on Bone Density in Osteoporotic Patients. Biomed Res Int. 2018;2018:4840531. Published 2018 Dec 23.

Information on astronauts

https://www.nasa.gov/mission_pages/station/research/benefits/bone_loss.html

Joel S. Finkelstein, Sarah E. Brockwell, Vinay Mehta, Gail A. Greendale, MaryFran R. Sowers, Bruce Ettinger, Joan C. Lo, Janet M. Johnston, Jane A. Cauley, Michelle E. Danielson, Robert M. Neer, Bone Mineral Density Changes during the Menopause Transition in a Multiethnic Cohort of Women, The Journal of Clinical Endocrinology & Metabolism, Volume 93, Issue 3, 1 March 2008, Pages 861–868,

Maltais, Mathieu & Desroches, J & Dionne, Isabelle. (2009). Changes in muscle mass and strength after menopause. Journal of musculoskeletal & neuronal interactions. 9. 186-97.

Cussler EC, Lohman TG, Going SB, Houtkooper LB, Metcalfe LL, Flint-Wagner HG, Harris RB, Teixeira PJ. Weight lifted in strength training predicts bone change in postmenopausal women. Med Sci Sports Exerc. 2003 Jan;35(1):10-7.

R.C. Offer, MD, FRCPC, FACR S.W. Offer, BSN Osteoporosis and Menopause; BCMJ, vol. 43 , No. 8 , October 2001 , Pages 458-462 Clinical Articles

Flynn CA. Calcium supplementation in postmenopausal women. Am Fam Physician. 2004 Jun 15;69(12):2822-3. PMID: 15222645.

Skin

Shah MG, Maibach HI. Estrogen and skin. An overview. Am J Clin Dermatol. 2001;2(3):143-50. doi: 10.2165/00128071-200102030-00003. PMID: 11705091.

Liu, T, Li, N, Yan, Y, et al. Recent advances in the anti-aging effects of phytoestrogens on collagen, water content, and oxidative stress. Phytotherapy Research. 2020; 34: 435– 447.

M. Julie Thornton (2013) Estrogens and aging skin, Dermato-Endocrinology, 5:2, 264-270, DOI: 10.4161/derm.23872

Eyes

Mark B. Abelson, MD, and Lisa Lines Hormones in Dry-Eye: A Delicate Balance Review of Ophthalmology 23 Feb 2006

Krenzer, Kathleen & Dana, M & Ullman, M & Cermak, Jennifer & Tolls, D & Evans, James & Sullivan, David. (2001). Effect of Androgen Deficiency on the Human Meibomian Gland and Ocular Surface. The Journal of clinical endocrinology and metabolism. 85. 4874-82. 10.1210/jc.85.12.4874.

Gut

Moderate Exercise Has Limited but Distinguishable Effects on the Mouse Microbiome American Society of Microbiology Emily V. Lamoureux, Scott A. Grandy, Morgan G. I. Langille

Yasmine Belkaid and Timothy Hand Role of the Microbiota in Immunity and inflammation Cell. 2014 March 27; 157(1): 121–141.

Barbara J. Fuhrman, Heather Spencer Feigelson, Roberto Flores, Mitchell H. Gail, Xia Xu, Jacques Ravel, James J. Goedert, Associations of the Fecal Microbiome With Urinary Estrogens and Estrogen Metabolites in Postmenopausal Women, The Journal of Clinical Endocrinology & Metabolism, Volume 99, Issue 12, December 2014, Pages 4632–4640

Duszka K, Wahli W. Enteric Microbiota–Gut–Brain Axis from the Perspective of Nuclear Receptors. International Journal of Molecular Sciences. 2018; 19(8):2210. (most interesting paper ever!)

207

Flores, R., Shi, J., Fuhrman, B. et al. Fecal microbial determinants of fecal and systemic estrogens and estrogen metabolites: a cross-sectional study. J Transl Med 10, 253 (2012).

Kristina B. Martinez, Vanessa Leone & Eugene B. Chang (2017) Western diets, gut dysbiosis, and metabolic diseases: Are they linked?, Gut Microbes, 8:2, 130-142

The Clever Guts Diet - Dr Michael Mosley

Fatigue

Taylor-Swanson L, Wong AE, Pincus D, et al. The dynamics of stress and fatigue across menopause: attractors, coupling, and resilience. Menopause. 2018;25(4):380-390. doi:10.1097/GME.0000000000001025

Chedraui P, Aguirre W, Hidalgo L, Fayad L. Assessing menopausal symptoms among healthy middle aged women with the Menopause Rating Scale. Maturitas. 2007;57(3):271–278.

Printed in Great Britain
by Amazon